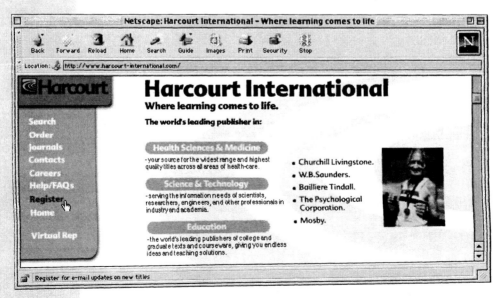
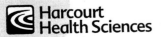

Managing Risk in Community Practice

Dedication

In loving memory of
Danuta Maria Alaszewski 1918–1997
Brenda Walker 1925–1991
Tess Manthorpe 1920–1975

For Baillière Tindall:

Senior Commissioning Editor: Jacqueline Curthoys
Project Development Manager: Karen Gilmour
Project Manager: Derek Robertson
Design Direction: George Ajayi

Managing Risk in Community Practice

Nursing, Risk and Decision Making

Andy Alaszewski BA PhD
Professor of Health Studies; Director, Institute of Health Studies, University of Hull, Hull, UK

Helen Alaszewski BA RGN
Research Assistant, School of Community and Health Studies, University of Hull, Hull, UK

Sam Ayer PhD BSc RN RNT FRSH CertEd
Senior Lecturer, School of Nursing, University of Hull, Hull, UK

Jill Manthorpe MA
Senior Lecturer, Department of Social Work, University of Hull, Hull, UK

Foreword by
Bob Heyman
Professor of Health Research, St. Bartholmew School of Nursing and Midwifery,
City University, London

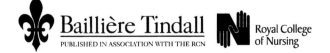

Baillière Tindall
PUBLISHED IN ASSOCIATION WITH THE RCN

Royal College
of Nursing

EDINBURGH LONDON NEW YORK PHILADELPHIA ST LOUIS SYDNEY TORONTO 2000

BAILLIÈRE TINDALL
An imprint of Harcourt Publishers Limited

© Harcourt Publishers Limited 2000

✤ is a registered trademark of Harcourt Publishers Limited

The right of Andy Alaszewski, Helen Alaszewski, Sam Ayer and Jill
Manthorpe to be identified as authors of this work has been asserted
by them in accordance with the Copyright, Designs and Patents Act
1988

First published 2000

ISBN 07020 2603 4

British Library Cataloguing in Publication Data
A catalogue record for this book is available from the British Library

Library of Congress Cataloging in Publication Data
A catalog record for this book is available from the Library of
Congress

Note
Medical knowledge is constantly changing. As new information
becomes available, changes in treatment, procedures, equipment and
the use of drugs become necessary. The authors and the publishers
have taken care to ensure that the information given in this text is
accurate and up-to-date. However, readers are strongly advised to
confirm that the information, especially with regard to drug usage,
complies with the latest legislation and standards of practice.

Printed and bound by Antony Rowe Ltd, Eastbourne

Contents

Contributors

Andy Alaszewski is Professor of Health Studies and Director of the Institute of Health Studies at the University of Hull. He has been an active researcher since 1972. His main research interests include the development of services for people with a learning disability, and risk assessment and management of health services. He has published extensively in academic and professional journals and is the author or editor of six books, including *Risk, Health and Welfare*, Open University Press, 1998; he is also editor of the international academic journal, *Health, Risk and Society*, published by Taylor and Francis.

Helen Alaszewski is a research assistant in the Institute of Health Studies. She is a qualified nurse who specialised in the care of older people before moving into nursing research. She remains committed to the development of clinical practice. She has undertaken research on discharge planning for older people and communication between hospital and residential homes and was the research assistant on the ENB-funded project into Risk Assessment and Management in Multi-Agency, Multi-Professional Care (1 February 1996 to 31 January 1998).

Sam Ayer is a Senior Lecturer in the School of Nursing and Director of Post-Graduate Education in the Faculty of Health at the University of Hull. He is a qualified nurse who specialised in learning disability and mental health nursing before moving into nursing education and research. His recent published work includes 'Services for People with Learning Disabilities' and 'Issue of Race and Ethnicity in Learning Disability,' in Gates, B. and Beacock, C. (eds) *Dimensions of Learning Disability*, Baillière Tindall, Edinburgh, 1997.

Jill Manthorpe is a Senior Lecturer in Community Care at the University of Hull. She has recently conducted research in the area of community care management, on risk and welfare services and the impact of local government reorganisation. Her publications include recent articles on care management, social work education, risk policies and dementia and contributions to books on social work, elder abuse, carers and learning disabilities. She is a Trustee of Action on Elder Abuse and has served as a Non-Executive Director of a local Community Health Trust.

Foreword

Citizens of 21st century, technologically driven societies are, collectively, as preoccupied with risk as their medieval ancestors were with God and religion. It is not surprising, therefore, that the 'new nursing' has made risk a central concern, documented in the UKCC *Guidelines for Mental Health and Learning Disability Nursing* (1998), as this timely, well-written book points out.

Although nurses will focus primarily on the welfare of their clients, they should also be able to reflect on the conceptual underpinnings of their work. A critical approach to risk throws up a number of puzzling questions. Even the meaning of the term is problematic. Are risks, for example, natural phenomena which, like diseases, can be observed, classified and measured, or, at the other end of the scale, entirely subjective? Why are societies like ours so concerned about risk? Why are some risks, for example, that a child will be murdered, treated as intolerable, whilst others, for instance, the risk that a child will be killed in a traffic accident, are coolly accepted? What does risk orientation imply for relationships between practitioners, including nurses, service users and unpaid, usually family, carers? *Managing Risk in Community Practice* raises such questions in an accessible way, linking them to analysis of the role of nurses in risk management for older people, people with learning disabilities and people with mental health problems.

Nurses concerned with risk management for vulnerable clients must confront the central dilemma of autonomy versus safety. As one client with learning difficulties quoted in the book puts it: 'there was a sand dune - it was hard to get up …. It was a risky thing but worth it. Someone was with us'. Although skilled and appropriate support, as in the example quoted, may minimise the price, in terms of risk of harm, of any given degree of autonomy, trade-offs cannot be avoided in risk management.

This dilemma takes a particularly sharp from for people whose health or other problems limit their ability to self-manage risk. The client groups discussed in this group are more likely than average to harm themselves and also more likely to be threatened by others. (Despite current political preoccupations in the UK, there is little evidence that members of the public are more likely to be harmed by people with serious mental health problems than they are by anyone else.)

Members of the client group discussed in the book often face complex combinations of disabilities and health problems which greatly complicate risk management. For example, one family carer of a diabetic young man with a learning disability found that when he visited friends they would give him tea with sugar, putting him at risk (see Chapter 3). Because of his learning disability, or perhaps because of the passivity which stigmatisation of this role induces, he did not ask his friends to give him sugarless tea. His parents were faced with the dilemma of curtailing his social activity versus accepting a serious health risk. This example, along with many others discussed in the book, clearly illustrates the need for skilled nursing support which helps clients and carers to manage risk/autonomy dilemma.

Dilemmas, by definition, cannot be managed in a single optimum way. Instead, a range of solutions which offer different balances, in this case between autonomy and safety, need to be considered. In the absence of a gold standard, nurses' contributions to risk management must take account, as appropriate, of the aspirations and beliefs of clients and family carers. The latter will have their own clear ideas about acceptable risk and will simply reject professional advice which does not acknowledge their own risk management strategies. And, as the book well illustrates, risks will often be seen from different perspectives. Professionals have to worry about the risk of litigation and of career damage. They are socialised into viewing risk in particular ways. The books draws a telling comparison between current mental health rhetoric which emphasises prevention of both risk to the public and of self-harm, and the ideology prevalent in the learning disabilities field which emphasises the value of autonomy and normalisation.

Given that risk management always involves selective attention to some contingencies rather than others, nurses need to develop sensitive asking and listening skills if they are to appreciate the perspectives of clients and family carers (see Chapter 3). One service user with a disability felt that the biggest risk at college was 'being ignored'. An older man was most worried that his wife would have to go into a Home if his health deteriorated. A carer associated the word 'risk' with professionals coming into her home!

The latter part of the book draws out implications of the preceding analysis for nurses' decision-making at both individual and organisational levels. It offers nurses an invaluable guide to the complex issues underlying a central aspect of their modern role, and will serve them well for many year to come.

Bob Heyman, 2000

Preface

Risk has become a central issue in the provision of health and welfare. In England health ministers are no longer willing to accept professional assurances that they can regulate their own practice and decision making. Through clinical governance, they have made the chief executives of health agencies responsible for the quality of professionals' decision making, identifying harmful practice and practitioners and the overall management of risk by their agency.

I first became aware of the importance of risk in community practice in the mid-1980s when I was undertaking an evaluative study of a community-based unit run by Barnardo's. The agency was committed to empowering children with profound learning disabilities by enabling them to experience ordinary living and the risks associated with it. However, it was clear that there were problems in achieving this desirable objective. The children had serious difficulties in communicating, which made it difficult to identify what they enjoyed and thus enable them to make choices. Some of the children were 'medically fragile', so the care staff and unit managers had to balance issues of safety against those of choice. The unit was not only home for the children but it was also a place of work and there was a need to take into account health and safety considerations. The unit was located in a new residential area so Barnardo's had to decide how much information to give neighbours. It is now clear to me that these issues were linked. They all involved assessing and managing some form of risk.

Although nurses' role as risk assessors and managers is now well established and accepted, I became concerned in the mid-1990s that risk was being defined in such a narrow and restricted way that there was a danger that nurses would be seen as some form of community police force, concerned primarily with controlling dangerous or threatening behaviours. I was pleased when the English National Board for Nursing, Midwifery and Health Visiting announced in 1995 that it was funding a major review of the education and practice of nurses providing support for vulnerable individuals living within the community. I was delighted when the ENB agreed to fund a team at the University of Hull to undertake this work. The team included me, Jill Manthorpe, Sam Ayer and Helen Alaszewski as the researcher.

While this book draws on that review, it is not a research report. That was published by the ENB (Alaszewski *et al.*, 1998a). We see this book as a key text for nurse education; it provides practising nurses, nurse lecturers and nursing students with an accessible guide to risk assessment and risk management in clinical practice, especially when caring and supporting vulnerable individuals in the community.

We start this book by considering why risk is an issue and in particular the importance of risk management in developing a relationship of trust between nurses, the users of their services and the general public. In the second chapter we develop this analysis by considering the tensions and ambiguities which nurses need to be aware of and resolve in their practice. In particular, we identify a tension between a restricted approach to risk, with a preoccupation with danger and harm, and a broader approach that acknowledges both danger and harm but balances them against more positive objectives such as user empowerment. It is important that nurses take into account the ways in which users and carers define risk and we explore their definitions in Chapter 3.

In the second part of the book we examine how nurses manage risk and in particular how it influences their decision making. In Chapter 4 we explore the issues in relationship to individual practice while in Chapter 5 we extend our analysis to consider the influence of team work on risk and decision making. In Chapter 6 we consider the education and professional developmental processes which can be used to enhance nurses' ability to manage risk and make decisions. In the final chapter we return to our opening theme of risk and trust and explore the ethical principles and values which should underpin risk assessment and management in nursing.

Andy Aleszewski, 2000

Acknowledgements

The research on which this book is based was commissioned by the English National Board for Nursing, Midwifery and Health Visiting who provided funding for the research team from 1 February 1996 until 31 January 1998.

We should like to thank the members of the Steering Group for their support, constructive criticism and guidance throughout the 2 years of the project and in particular Jane Keithley who chaired the meetings and Sonia Crow who took a close and sustained interest in our research.

We also wish to express our gratitude to the numerous educationalists, students and practitioners who participated in and contributed to the project. We would like to thank the members of the user and carer groups and all those who provided assistance from the Faculty of Health where we are based. We are unable to acknowledge the contribution of the participants in the research personally as we have used pseudonyms to ensure anonymity.

This book draws on research to illustrate key issues in the ways in which nurses assess and manage risk. While it is not a research report, the book builds upon the insights of our ENB-funded research. The ENB has already published a research report in its researching professional education series (Alaszewski *et al.*, 1998a). We have taken the opportunity provided by this book to develop our analysis and examining its relevance to contemporary nurse education and practice. Readers who wish to have a fuller account of the research methodology and of educational issues should consult this report. We thank the ENB for giving us permission to utilise some of the material published in the report and we also thank the UKCC for its permission to reproduce material from its various publications.

Risk in nursing practice: developing and sustaining trust

Andy Alaszewski

INTRODUCTION

In health and welfare services there are fads and fashions. In the 1970s nurses were encouraged to identify and meet clients' and patients' needs; in the 1980s they were expected to provide quality services to consumers or customers; and today they are expected to protect users, themselves and the public from risk, danger and harm. In this chapter we examine the nature of risk in current society and nursing practice and the importance of trust as the basis for risk management.

THE RISE OF RISK

Risk is a modern concept and word. In the English language the word was first used in the 17th century and was derived from the French word *risque*, which in turn was derived from Italian *risco* (for a discussion of the origins see Ayto, 1990: 446, and Wharton, 1992).

Initially, risk was associated with gaming and gambling and attracted the intellectual curiosity of contemporary thinkers. In the 1650s the mathematicians

Pascal and Fermat developed the basis of the modern theory of probability by studying intellectual puzzles such as how two players fairly should share the stakes of an uncompleted game of chance (Bernstein, 1996: 57–62). With the decline of religion and the explanation of events and actions in religious terms, such as the will of God or fate, so explanations of events and actions in terms of risk have become increasingly important (Giddens, 1990). Indeed Beck (1992) has argued that risk has become a central feature and issue within modern industrial society and has referred to contemporary society as *risk society*. Given the importance of health and welfare within modern society, it is hardly surprising that risk should feature prominently in debates about health and welfare. As Adams points out, it is impossible to read a modern newspaper or watch the television news and not come across a story involving risk:

> *Consider an ordinary news day chosen at random – 28 January 1994, the day this sentence was written. A perusal of that day's papers reveals that the business sections and the sports pages contain virtually no stories that are not about the management of risk. They are all about winning and losing, the winners and losers. The heroes are people who struggled against the odds and won …. The health pages were of course entirely devoted to risk stories: a chickenpox vaccine whose effectiveness remains to be proven; a series of mistakes in cervical cancer screening that 'put patients' lives at risk' … the fear that bovine spongiform encephalopathy might have spread to humans in the form of Creutzfeld–Jacob disease.* (Adams, 1995: 2).

Saunders, in his review of risk in services for people with a learning disability, notes the importance of risk in the following way:

> *If importance were measured in terms of the degree to which an issue was raised and discussed at all levels within a service, then risk management would have few peers. Within the context of service delivery to people with a learning disability the term risk management is never too far removed from the lips of service professionals and service managers alike.* (Saunders, 1999: 13).

Like many of the key words in health and social care, risk has a variety of meanings and these can create confusion and ambiguity (for an analysis of another key word, quality, see Alaszewski and Manthorpe, 1993).

Douglas (1990) argued that the original meaning of risk was associated with chance and consequence:

> *The concept originally emerged in the seventeenth century in the context of gambling. For this purpose a specialised mathematical analysis of chances was developed. Risk then meant the probability of an event occurring, combined with the magnitude of the losses or gains that would be entailed.* (Douglas, 1990: 2).

This balance of potential negative consequences of events and actions with desired positive outcomes can be seen in early definitions. For example, in 1759, Dr Johnson used risk in the sense of balancing gain against loss:

> *To risque the certainty of little for the chance of much.* (Cited in Simpson and Weiner, 1989: 988).

One quotation which Johnson used in his dictionary to illustrate contemporary usage, defined risk in terms of the balance between potential loss and gain:

> *Some run the risk of an absolute ruin for the gaining of a present supply.* (Quote from *L'Etrange's Fable*, Johnson, 1775, cited in Simpson and Weiner, 1989: 988).

However, from its earliest introduction into the English language, the everyday use of risk has emphasised its negative elements and risk has been defined as the negative consequences of an event or action. For example, Blount, in his glossography published in 1661 lists 'peril, jeopardy, danger, hazard, and chance' as synonyms for *risque* (cited in Simpson and Weiner, 1989: 987). This emphasis remains prominent in the everyday usage of risk. Current dictionary definitions emphasise the negative aspects equating risk with danger, harm and loss. For example the *New Oxford Dictionary of English* provides the following definition of risk and illustrations of the contemporary use of risk as a noun:

> *a situation involving exposure to danger:* flouting the law was too much of a risk/all outdoor activities carry an element of risk .... (Normal type was in italics in the original, Pearsall, 1998: 1602).

and as a verb:

> *expose (someone or something valued) to danger, harm, or loss:* he risked his life to save his dog ....
> *incur the chance of unfortunate consequences by engaging in (an action).* (Normal type was italics in the original, Pearsall, 1998: 1602).

Thus, risk is frequently identified with threat to an individual or a group which can result in harm, loss or negative consequences. Risk is often used interchangeably with hazard or a danger (see Warner, 1992: p. 4 for a discussion of hazard).

This emphasis on the negative aspect of risk is also evident in more specialist literature. Dobos, in a study of nurses' perspectives of risk, defined risk as

> *any situation in which the outcome is uncertain and in which something of value could be lost.* (Dobos, 1992: 1304).

While in a study of risk and mental health nursing, Ryan noted:

> *The way that risk has been defined to date in mental health has largely been to do with physical harm to self or others.* (Ryan, 1999: xiv).

Within contemporary definitions, it is possible to identify an alternative approach which can be linked to earlier definitions of risk as the probability of either positive or negative outcomes. For example, one of the definitions provided in the *New Oxford Dictionary of English* of risk as a noun is

> *a person or thing regarded as likely to turn out well or badly, as specified, in a particular context or respect:* Western banks regarded Romania as a good risk. (Pearsall, 1998: 1602).

This approach can also be identified in the more technical literature and usage. For example, Wharton, an expert in operational research, employed a definition which explicitly avoids evaluating the value of the unexpected outcome:

> *A risk is an unintended or unexpected outcome of a decision or course of action.* (Wharton, 1992: 2).

Nonetheless, there are also approaches to risk which give particular prominence to its positive aspects. These approaches tend to focus on the benefits to be gained from the process of taking risks. This type of approach is well illustrated in Pritchard's discussion of 'vulnerable people taking risks':

> *We all take risks to achieve something we want and in many situations we experience various emotions whilst taking the risk – enjoyment, excitement, fear, anxiety. If we achieve what we want, we then experience a great sense of achievement and fulfilment and we may get approval and respect from others.* (Pritchard, 1997: 81).

Alberg *et al.* (1996) in their learning materials on mental health define risk in terms of consequences and probability:

> *So Risk can be seen as having two components:*
>
> 1. *The types of harm and benefits that may arise*
> 2. *The likelihood of those harms and benefits arising.* (Alberg et al., 1996: 9).

Since health and welfare services are usually concerned with achieving certain specified outcomes, our preferred definition would also include the concept of intention and for the purposes of this book we define risk as

> *the possibility that a given course of action will not achieve its desired and intended outcome but instead some unintended situation will develop.* (adapted from Alaszewski and Manthorpe, 1991: 277).

Box 1.1 Elements underlying risk

◆ The consequences of actions.

◆ The probability of different types of consequences.

◆ The intentions of the individuals involved.

Underlying this definition of risk are three interrelated elements (Box 1.1). Different individuals and groups may use different definitions of risk and we will explore in Chapters 2 and 3 the implications of the varying definitions held by nurses, service users and informal carers. In the remainder of this chapter we will explore the importance of risk in the provision of health care in general and nursing in particular.

TRUSTING EXPERTS

Individuals and social groups in all societies have to cope with threats posed to their health and well-being by natural processes such as earthquakes and disease and man-made events such as war. However, social and techno-logical developments have changed both the nature of these threats and the mechanisms used to cope with them. Prior to the development of large-scale urban societies associated with the industrial revolution, societies were small scale and based on highly personalised relations. In many parts of the world these types of social relations persist and have been studied by anthropologists.

From the perspective of modern science the response in these societies to both individual and group threats such as ill health or death is irrational, as the threats are explained in supernatural terms such as witchcraft or sorcery. However, anthropologists argue that individuals in these traditional societies are as rational as individuals in modern societies (Leach, 1957: 129): they understand and use appropriate technologies to protect themselves. However, given the limitations of available technologies, individuals need additional ways of explaining and controlling natural and social events, especially abnormal or threatening events that threaten individual or group security. These threats are interpreted as interventions by gods, spirits, witches and sorcerers in natural and social events, and such societies developed explanations and expertise so that they could manage these interventions. As Lupton has noted, there was a similar situation in medieval France where both peasants and aristocrats were vulnerable to many threats to their health and lives and:

magic, combined with a dash of Christianity, served as the belief system by which threats and dangers were dealt with conceptually and behaviourally, allowing people to feel that they had some control over their world.
(Lupton, 1999: 2).

In many earlier societies, experts in the supernatural both provided explanations of and protections against the misfortunes of life. For example, 'witch doctors' have the skills and expertise to identify witches and counteract their malevolent influence (for a classic anthropological account, see Evans-Pritchard, 1937). As nurses will be aware, scientists' clear differentiation between rational and irrational explanations of events in modern societies is not necessarily shared by lay people, who mix 'scientific' and 'nonscientific' elements together in their explanations for misfortunes such as illness (Leach, 1957: 129; for an account of 'irrational' lay explanations of ill health in modern society, see Helman, 1994).

Modern societies are characterised by the development of sophisticated technologies based on scientific research that have enabled them to exert control over their environment and to provide increased security and welfare. These technologies are used by experts employed by large, often state-funded, bureaucracies to provide individual citizens with welfare and protection. In modern societies:

Rational thinking, bureaucratic systems of prevention, ways of identifying threats before they take effect, are regularly put forward as means of managing danger and threats. (Lupton, 1999: 3–4).

The National Health Service uses medical technologies, such as vaccinations and radiography, to reduce threats such as infectious diseases and increase our ability to intervene within the body, and these technologies have been associated with increased life expectancies (Giddens, 1991: 115–18). However, since the technologies which underpin such developments are beyond the scope of understanding of most individuals in modern society, they are also associated with a 'fright' or 'fear' factor so that subjective assessments of risk often exceed objective assessments. Calman and his colleagues (Calman *et al.*, 1999: 111) identified a number of fright factors which increase awareness and fear of risk. These fright factors tend to be linked to the very technologies which experts present as 'safe' and beneficial. These are often experienced as 'threatening', because they act invisibly and are difficult to understand; 'disempowering', because they remove control from the individual; and 'unfair', because they harm the most vulnerable individuals in society (see Box 1.2).

Beck also pointed out that modern technology is threatening because its effects are not localised. Technological change affects the whole globe and

---

Box 1.2 Fright factors (factors associated with increased subjective perception of threat) (adapted from Calman et al., 1999: 111)

Individual and group perception of threat is increased if threat is associated with:

new technology

◆ results from man-made, rather than natural sources

◆ arises from unfamiliar or novel sources.

loss of individual control

◆ to be involuntary, e.g. exposure to pollution rather than voluntary, e.g. dangerous sport or smoking

◆ to cause hidden and irreversible damage, e.g through onset of illness many years after exposure, e.g. effects of radiation

◆ to threaten a form of death, or illness/injury, arousing particular dread, such as cancer.

lack of information

◆ to be poorly understood by science, such as HIV/AIDS in the 1980s

◆ as subject to contradictory statements from responsible sources, or, even worse, from the same source, such as BSE in the early stages.

unfairness

◆ as inequitably distributed, some benefit while others suffer the consequences

◆ to pose some particular danger to small children or pregnant women or more generally to future generations

◆ to damage identifiable rather than anonymous victims.

---

major technological catastrophes such as the Chernobyl nuclear accident have the capacity to invisibly affect everywhere:

> It is … *striking that hazards in those days [Middle Ages in Europe] assaulted the nose or the eyes and were thus perceptible to the senses, while the risks of civilization today typically* escape perception *and are localized in the sphere of* physical and chemical formulas *(e.g. toxins in foodstuffs or the nuclear threat)* …. *[Modern risks] are risks* of modernization. *They are a* wholesale product *of industrialization, and are systematically intensified as it becomes global.* (Normal type shows emphases in the original; Beck, 1992: 21).

However, this perception of a global disaster is not a new phenomenon: just as some individuals feared the start of the new millennium would result in a major global disaster, so many Christians expected that the first millennium would end with Armageddon and the end of the world. The difference is the anticipated cause of the disaster: divine intervention at the end of the first millennium and the man-made millennium bug spread through hidden technology at the end of the second millennium.

Giddens has argued that all societies perceive threats and that they seek to maintain order and security by counteracting such threats. He referred to such threats as 'risk', using the terms of negative consequences: i.e. threats to individual and collective well-being and security. He contrasted it to 'trust', which he saw as a way of providing individuals and groups with security and counteracting the threats posed by risk. Indeed, Giddens saw trust as a 'protective cocoon' which provided individuals with security by filtering out the 'potential dangers impinging from the external world'. (Giddens 1991: 244).

Trust is not an optional extra; it is an essential part of individual development. Giddens has stated that:

> *Learning the characteristics of absent friends and objects – accepting the real world as real – depends on the emotional security that basic trust provides. The feeling of unreality which may haunt the lives of individuals in whose early childhood trust was poorly developed may take many forms. They may feel that the object-world, or other people, have only a shadow existence, or be unable to maintain a clear sense of continuity of self-identity.* (Giddens, 1991: 43).

It can also be demonstrated that trust has a therapeutic effect. For example, the development of trust between nurses and surgical patients through the provision of information about the nature and consequences of surgery has measurable beneficial therapeutic effects in reducing pain (Hayward, 1975). The harm experienced by children deprived of a trusting relationship was well documented in the 1940s and 1950s. For example, in 1956 the Chief Medical Officer of Health of the Ministry of Health commented adversely on the effects of institutional care on children arguing that they needed:

> *love, security, companionship and stimulation if the personality is to develop normally.* (cited in Shearer, 1980: 53).

Giddens (1990: 100–11) argued that modernity does not create risk and trust, but it changes their nature. Traditional societies tend to be highly localised in terms of social, political and economic relations. Risk and trust are also localised and personalised with strong emphasis on individual relations of trust. Family and kin live in close proximity and provide individuals with a sense of security. Individuals in premodern society use their personal knowledge to establish relationships of trust; they use their personal knowledge of their kin or local experts to evaluate their trustworthiness. Modernisation disrupts these highly personalised and localised relations. The extended localised kin networks of premodern society have been replaced by a more variable mix of immediate family and friends which is both less reliable and can only provide limited support and expertise. In modern societies, when individuals have to deal with serious threats· which require major resources and expertise they normally have to rely on the impersonal support provided by welfare agencies and welfare professionals. Thus, in modern society, transactions involving highly sensitive and potentially damaging information and necessitating access to intimate parts of an individual's life and body, such as the diagnosis and treatment of disease, often take place between strangers. Paradoxically, the greater the threat to our well-being the more we are dependant on the skills, expertise and goodwill of strangers (Giddens, 1990: 84).

It is possible to deal with such encounters by treating them as if they were based on a traditional face-to-face relationship. For example, in the British National Health Service, general medical practitioners are called 'family practitioners' and there is an implication that they will have a personal knowledge of each member of the family. However, when individual users cannot rely on such personal knowledge then they require other guarantees. They need to be reassured that the decisions made are not only made with appropriate expertise but also in their interest (Giddens, 1990: 85). This is particularly important when the decisions are fateful and involve major and irreversible changes in people's lives:

> Fateful moments *are those when individuals are called on to make decisions that are particularly consequential for their ambitions, or more generally for their future lives. Fateful moments are highly consequential for a person's destiny.* (Normal type shows emphasis in the original, Giddens, 1991: 112).

Giddens was concerned with decisions made by individuals themselves, but in some circumstances professionals must make these decisions on behalf of vulnerable individuals. However, as Giddens pointed out, even when individuals do make these decisions, because of their high consequences and uncertainty, they are likely to draw on expert advice:

> *Fateful moments, or rather that category of possibilities which an individual defines as fateful, stand in a particular relation to risk …. Experts are often brought in as a fateful moment approaches or a fateful decision has to be taken. Quite commonly, in fact, expertise is the vehicle whereby a particular circumstance is pronounced as fateful, as for instance in the case of a*

medical diagnosis .... Fateful decisions are usually almost by definition difficult to take because of the mixture of the problematic and the consequential that characterises them. (Giddens, 1991: 113–14).

Thus, in modern society, individuals have to depend on and trust experts, especially when they are involved in fateful decisions. In the next section, we explore the growing concerns about the trustworthiness of experts.

PROFESSIONALS, TRUST AND DECISIONS

At the high point of professional development in Britain in the 1950s, there was unconditional trust by both politicians and the public in professional decision making and professional judgement. Thus, the growth of the welfare state in the 1950s involved not only a substantial increase in public expenditure on health and welfare but the delegation of control of this expenditure to professional groups. Indeed, Rhodes (1987: 101) described the post-war period as the 'era of the professional'. Since the 1950s there has been a loss of confidence in professionals, especially by the state. The inexorable rise of state expenditure on welfare and the recessions of the 1980s placed a strain on the relationship between the state and professionals and there is no longer an automatic acceptance of professional decision making and judgements (see, for example, Dowie & Elstein, 1988a). As Cook and Easthope (1996: 86) point out:

like other expert systems, the institution of medicine is having to contend with diminishing trust on the part of all those who come into contact with, or work within such institutions.

Early analysts of professions argued that professionals were 'trusted' to make important decisions on behalf of individuals and society as they had special expertise which they applied in a disinterested way. Talcott Parsons described the suitability of the professions in making key decisions such as allocating limited resources in terms of their 'collectivity-orientation' and contrasted it with the self-interest of the businessman in the following way:

the physician is a technically competent person whose competence and specific judgements and measures cannot be competently judged by the layman ... it would be particularly difficult to implement the pattern of the business world (for the delivery of medical care), where each party to the situation is expected to be oriented to the rational pursuit of his own self-interests, and where there is an approach to the idea of 'caveat emptor.' In a broad sense it is surely clear that society would not tolerate the privileges which have been vested in the medical profession on such terms. (Parsons, 1951: 463).

Parsons argued that the major expansion of professions that accompanied the growth of state activity in general and the welfare state in particular resulted in the development a new form of social structure. This structure has replaced both the political authoritarianism of premodern states and economic exploitation associated with markets dominated by capitalism in the 19th century:

> It (the professional complex) has displaced the 'state', in the relatively modern sense of that term, and, more recently, the 'capitalistic' organization of the economy. The massive emergence of the professional complex, not the special status of capitalistic or socialistic modes of organization, is the crucial structural development in twentieth-century society. (Parsons, 1966: 545).

Trust underpins a key and defining characteristic of professionals – their self-regulation. Professionals are not subjected to external regulation but are trusted to regulate their own affairs, especially the nature and quality of service received by the users of their services because they are trusted. Hanlon (1998: 48) sees trust as the central feature of the relationship between professionals and their employers. Trust is central to professional claims for self-regulation and forms an important part of their code of ethics or practice. For example, the UKCC's Code of Professional Conduct specified that:

> Each registered nurse, midwife and health visitor shall act, at all times, in such a manner as to...
>
> ◆ justify public trust and confidence and
> ◆ uphold and enhance the good standing and reputation of the professions. (UKCC, 1992).

Professions are finding it increasingly difficult to sustain the trust of the public and of governments. Their claims to special expertise are challenged by users of their services who challenge the view that professionals have all the relevant expertise while service users are ignorant. Users increasingly have access to alternative sources of information and expertise such as the internet and specialist helplines. Some practitioners are expressing concern that patients are accessing alternative expertise through the web (see Wyatt, 1998: 105). One patient who developed distressing symptoms indicating a progressive disease affecting his nerves described how he developed his own expertise and using it to educate 'ignorant' professionals:

> I woke at night and couldn't feel my forearms; as I moved there was a rush of blood, followed by terrible cramps in the muscles. By the end of the fifth week I was racked with pain. During this distressing time a friend noticed the BMJ article [on Lyme disease], did some research on Lyme disease, and suggested I

may have contracted it. I mentioned it to my GP, who was making an appointment for me to see a rheumatology specialist. The categorical answer came back from the consultant: there is no Lyme disease in the UK .... I checked on the World Wide Web and found LymeNet with a list of all the symptoms; it gave an almost perfect correlation [with my symptoms].

But was it in the UK? The web took me to EUCALB [and within] the space of a few minutes I had contacted the Lyme Disease Reference Unit at Southampton Public Health Laboratory. Doctors there agreed that my symptoms could match Lyme disease and said that I should immediately arrange for a blood sample to be sent to her [sic]. My GP was very helpful, two samples of blood were dispatched and 10 days later the results from the two stage test confirmed that I have Lyme disease. I am pleased that it is Lyme disease: if caught in the early stages it is easily treated with a course of antibiotics. (Spencer, 1997: 16).

As Hanlon points out:

[in the past] professionals supposedly provided solutions to a largely ignorant client base .... This ignorant client base may now be fundamentally changing in the light of Giddens' suggestion that one of the basic characteristics of high modernity is that individuals no longer simply 'trust' expert systems ... [people are encouraged] to question and learn from their interaction with society. (Hanlon, 1998: 50–1).

However, it is not just the expertise of professionals that is being challenged; it is also their claim to act ethically, that is for the general good. Professionals' claims to act in the public interest are no longer readily accepted. Adams examined the ways in which one group of professionals, engineers, balance self-interest and public interest. He noted that engineering disasters were seen as preventable:

Engineering disasters ... tend to be sudden and dramatic, involving collapse, collision, fire, explosion or escape of toxic substances. Inquests into engineering disasters, such as Piper Alpha, Zeebrugge and the Kings Cross fire, inevitably discover information which, had it been acted upon in time, would have averted the disaster. (Adams, 1995: 186).

Adams could find little evidence to indicate that engineers could be trusted to put public interest above their self or commercial interest. He analysed a paper presented by the chairman of the Fellowship of Engineers which described how the chairman issued a safety warning about an oil platform which was acted on by the platform owners and concluded that:

The impression that one gains from this account is that Good Samaritans willing to be drawn into responsibility for other people's safety problems are difficult to find in the engineering profession; that five weeks from suspicion of catastrophe to formal warning is an uncommonly brief period; that 'warners' agonize about the non-safety consequences of their warnings; and that 'warnees' prepared to bear the financial cost involved in doing the honourable thing are sufficiently rare to merit a strong sense of admiration. (Adams, 1995: 187–8).

This concern with disasters has resulted in the systematic analysis of 'man-made disasters'. Turner in his analysis of 'man-made disasters' defined a disaster as:

an event, concentrated in time and space, which threatens a society ... with major unwanted consequences as a result of the collapse of precautions which have hitherto been culturally accepted as adequate. (Turner and Pidgeon, 1997: 70).

Turner argued that such disasters indicated a failure in management and expertise. Gherardi applied the model to a major health disaster, the BSE (bovine spongiform encephalopathy) or mad cow disease. She pointed out that a key element in development of the disaster occurred during its 'incubation stage' when experts failed to realise the significance of information which would have provided a warning:

The BSE disease as a new neurological disease was identified in the mid-1980s and epidemiological studies completed. At that time BSE was just a 'science story'. The inference was that scrapie (the encephalopathy of sheep) had crossed the species barrier via cattle food supplements containing sheep carcasses. Alarms sounded in scientific circles that another jump – from cows to people through beef eating – was possible. But the division of labour in science kept veterinary and human medicine separate and the risk of the BSE agent crossing the boundaries was underestimated. (Gherardi, 1999: 237–8).

Although natural disasters and man-made disasters may have different causes, it is important to note that the harmful consequences of natural disasters can and are substantially amplified by human actions. The design and construction of safety systems by experts can create a false sense of security. For example, the *Titanic*, was designed to be unsinkable; when it hit an iceberg, it did not have enough liferafts for all the crew and passengers.

Although disasters draw attention to failure in the ways experts use information and make decisions, researchers studying professional decision making under 'normal' conditions have also identified problems in terms of both the process of decision making and its outcomes. A major concern is that professionals, such as doctors, when they are given the same information often make very different decisions:

The wide variation in clinical practices uncovered by virtually all studies of clinical behaviour – whether the comparison is between colleagues, communities or countries – has been one empirical focus for those attempting to assess professional performance. The significant percentage of discrepancies between clinical diagnoses and pathological findings which emerges in most autopsy studies is another. (Dowie and Elstein, 1988a: 2).

To achieve better outcomes, Eddy argues that practitioners should use information more effectively and that they should handle the uncertainty of decision making by using decision support techniques:

Over the past few hundred years languages have developed for collecting and interpreting evidence (statistics), dealing with uncertainty (probability theory), synthesizing evidence and estimating outcomes (mathematics), and making decisions (economics and decision theory). These languages are not currently learned by most clinical policymakers; they should be. (Eddy, 1988: 58).

The government's response to this evidence has been to seek to develop more systematic decision making. In the National Health Service, this has involved the development of clinical guidelines and the use of evidence-based practice. This move to greater central control of professional decision making underpins the government's White Paper on the NHS:

In a changing world no organisation, however great, can stand still. The NHS needs to modernise in order to meet the demands of today's public. This White Paper begins the process of modernisation. (Department of Health, 1997b: 3).

Central to this programme of modernisation is the collection and use of scientific knowledge as the basis of decision making to ensure the most effective and efficient delivery of health care. In the White Paper three separate mechanisms are identified to ensure knowledge will be used in the NHS.

◆ National Service Frameworks. *The Government will work with professionals and representatives to establish clearer, evidence-based National Service Frameworks for major care area and disease groups. That way patients will get greater consistency in the availability and quality of services, right across the NHS;*
◆ National Institute for Clinical Excellence ... *will be established to give coherence and prominence to information about clinical and cost-effectiveness. It will produce and disseminate clinical guidelines based on relevant evidence of clinical and cost-effectiveness;*
◆ Commission for Health Improvement ... *will complement the introduction of clinical governance arrangements. [It] will offer an*

independent guarantee that local systems to monitor, assure and improve clinical quality are in place. (Department of Health, 1997b: 57–9).

This approach stresses the importance of knowledge but it fails to address directly the issue of how to use that knowledge to inform decisions which sustain and develop trust between the professional and the user.

MECHANISMS FOR ENHANCING TRUST

Trust is an elusive concept. It is about the personal character of relationships and, in particular, relationships in which the parties do not see the need for checks so that statements and claims can be accepted without additional evidence or questioning. It is easier to define trust negatively than positively. We become aware of its absence when something has gone wrong in a relationship: for example, when a parent kills his or her child or a teacher has a sexual relationship with an underage pupil. Trust is embedded within relationships. A relationship based on trust is one in which both parties accept a mutuality of interest and reliance. A trustworthy person is one who is what he or she appears to be, does what he or she says and maintains his or her part of an agreement. Thus in modern society the concept of trust is essentially projected from the known personal and intimate relationship onto unknown and impersonal relationships. For example, when Adams analysed the nature of risk and trust in modern society he moved from the highly personal relationship between a child and his or her parent to the impersonal relationship between citizens and the state:

> *Most decisions about risks involving infants and young children are taken by adults. Between infancy and adulthood there is a progressive handing over of responsibility. Adults are considered* responsible *for their actions, but they are not always considered trustworthy or sufficiently well informed. A third tier of responsibility [individual's own, parent for a child] consists of various* authorities *whose rôle with respect to adults is similar to that of adults with respect to children. The authorities are expected to be possessed of superior wisdom about the nature of risks and how to manage them.* (Adams, 1995: 2).

The second element of trust involves a 'taken for granted element'. When you trust someone or something you do not seek additional proof. You do not need to maintain controls or checks over a trustworthy person; once they have agreed to do something they will do it. Giddens has defined trust as:

> *The vesting of confidence in persons or abstract systems, made on the basis of a 'leap into faith' which brackets [filters out] ignorance or lack of information.* (Giddens, 1991: 244).

The taken for granted aspect of trust is particularly important in modern society. To manage our everyday lives we have to trust strangers. As Schutz has argued, we do this by using our 'common sense': that is, by using our understanding and knowledge of the typical and expected behaviours of individuals fulfilling defined roles. For example, if I trust the Royal Mail to deliver a letter which I post, then:

> *Putting a letter in the mailbox, I expect that unknown people, called postmen, will act in a typical way, not quite intelligible to me, with the result that my letter will reach the addressee within typically reasonable time.* (Schutz, 1971: 17).

As Schutz argues, the more anonymous the relationship, the more it has to be based on abstract generalisations:

> *In complete anonymization the individuals are supposed to be interchangeable and the course-of-action type refers to the behavior of 'whomsoever' acting in the way defined as typical by the construct.* (Schutz, 1971: 18).

A related point is made by Goffman in his discussion of stigma. He argued that when we first encounter strangers we make assumptions about their identity which includes judgments about their trustworthiness:

> *The routines of social intercourse in established settings allow us to deal with anticipated others without special attention or thought. When a stranger comes into our presence, then, first appearances are likely to enable us to anticipate his category and attributes, his 'social identity' – to use a term that is better than 'social status' because personal attributes such as 'honesty' are involved, as well as structural ones, like 'occupation'.* (Goffman, 1968: 12).

For Goffman, stigma is a characteristic of an individual which could discredit them and therefore make us doubt their trustworthiness. An individual who has a stigma is one who:

> *might have been received easily in ordinary social intercourse [but who] possesses a trait that can obtrude itself upon attention and turn those of us whom he meets away from him, breaking the claim that his other attributes have on us.* (Goffman, 1968: 15).

The challenge which stigma presents to an individual's claim to be trustworthy is clear in some of Goffman's examples of stigma:

> *blemishes of individual character perceived as weak will, domineering or unnatural passions, treacherous and rigid beliefs, and dishonesty, these*

Box 1.3 Examples of factors that influence perceptions

◆ The professional's classification of the type of user; for example, an habitual user of illicit drugs is not likely to be seen as trustworthy.

◆ The user's expectations of a specific occupation; for example, the Black community in London is not likely to see police constables employed by the metropolitan police force as trustworthy.

◆ Both parties' recollections of experience of previous similar encounters and especially encounters between the same individuals.

◆ The specific nature and character of the encounter.

being inferred from a known record of, for example, mental disorder, imprisonment, addiction, alcoholism, homosexuality, unemployment, suicidal attempts. (Goffman, 1968: 14).

Thus for a stranger to be trusted in the role of a doctor or nurse who has intimate access to our person and lives, we expect him or her not only to 'act the part' but also to 'look the part'.

The establishment and maintenance of trust within a specific relationship between a professional and a service user will be influenced by both the professionals' and the users' perceptions. These perceptions will be influenced by a number of factors (Box 1.3).

In modern society the general perceptions of 'typical' behaviours are heavily influenced by images and events recorded in the mass media. It is clear that these media events tend to portray occupations performing similar tasks in very different ways. For example, social workers have argued that the media representation of their activities is biased, with reporting that only focusses on their work with children and is overwhelmingly critical (Franklin, 1999).

This reflects the ways in which errors that undermine trust are dealt with. The medical profession which enjoys a high professional status has traditionally been allowed a high level of self-regulation. Accidents and incidents tend to be investigated by the profession itself using confidential inquiries: for example, homicides and suicides among psychiatric patients (Boyd, 1996). Social workers have not had a self-regulating system, although this is due to change with the announcement of the formation of a General Social Care Council (Department of Health, 1996). Social workers' errors are subject to both external review by inquiries and the media. Reder *et al.* (1993) have reviewed inquiry reports into child death as a result of carer abuse between 1973 and 1989. They conclude that although the intention of the panels was not to seek individual scapegoats, nevertheless 'there can be little doubt that discovering who was to blame dominated many of the panels' thinking' (Reder *et al.*, 1993: 135), and this blame has tended to fall upon fieldworkers (particularly social workers, but also health professionals) and their managers.

It is important to note that neither nurses nor doctors are immune to adverse media comment. This has particularly focussed on failures of professional self-regulation. As Gilbert has pointed out, bodies such as the United Kingdom Central Council for Nursing, Midwifery and Health Visiting (UKCC) and the General Medical Council are guardians of trust (Gilbert, 1998: 1015). However, there is a developing perception that the current system of self-regulation is failing to maintain the confidence of the public. The Secretary of State, Stephen Dorrell, initiated a review of the United Kingdom Central Council for Nursing, Midwifery and Health Visiting following a number of controversial decisions that enabled individuals who have betrayed the trust vested in them to practice as nurses. For example, the UKCC decided to restore several nurses convicted of rape to the Register (Coombes, 1999: 5). The Department of Health has noted that:

> *Recent events have dented public confidence in the quality of clinical care provided by the NHS.* (Department of Health, 1998b: para 3.44).

In the case of medicine, the preventable death of 29 children in Bristol Royal Infirmary was seen as a major disaster and resulted in a significant change in the regulatory process, with the General Medical Council taking a proactive role in ensuring that all doctors remain competent to practice (see Health Act, 1999, Schedule 3).

However, the key factors which shape users' perceptions of professions are their interactions with individual professionals. The importance of these interactions can be seen in situations where individuals have little opportunity to interact with experts who are making crucial decisions which affect them. This can be seen in the case of airline pilots. As Cox *et al.* (1992; 78–9) have pointed out, measured in fatalities per kilometre covered, the safest form of travel is by scheduled air service and two of the most dangerous forms of travel are walking and cycling. However, it is clear that individual perceptions of the danger of these forms of travel are very different. There is a well-established 'fear of flying', which relates to a number of factors. Walkers or cyclists use a simple technology that they both understand and control. Airline passengers use a complex technology that they neither control nor, in many cases, understand; furthermore, they rely on experts whom they neither know nor see, especially the aircrew and the pilot. They do not have the face-to-face contact through which they can judge the trustworthiness of the experts. Most airlines now encourage their pilots to talk to their passengers over the intercom system so that the pilots can establish some personal contact and reassure their passengers, thus reducing their fear and anxiety.

An interaction is not only likely to be influenced by previous experiences. The effects of a badly managed interaction which undermines the trust and confidence of the service user may be amplified. The interaction may become part of the user's narrative. It becomes a 'horror story' which through continual retelling can shape the perceptions of large numbers of service users, especially if the mass media picks up the story. Indeed, in our own research, several participants used 'horror stories' to illustrate their points and some of them we draw upon in our discussion of users' and carers' perceptions of risk management in Chapter 3.

A good interaction is one that reinforces the trust between those involved. This occurs when the participants feel that they are working together and sharing in the process of making decisions. Coote has argued that this trust can be developed through a genuine commitment by health and welfare agencies and the professionals they employ to openness and participation in decision making:

> *The mutual respect which is integral to an adult-to-adult relationship implies a degree of trust in the other. Not blind faith, but the kind of measured confidence that comes from informed understanding. Trust has broken down because politics is characterized by secrecy, spin-doctoring and special pleading. We can only rebuild it by moving forwards, not backwards .... A high-trust democracy is built on understanding and consensus not on instruction and obedience.* (Coote, 1998: 126).

Giddens argued that the general sense of powerlessness and anxiety which individuals in modern society experience (Giddens, 1991: 191–4) can be overcome if individuals question and if experts are willing and able to make explicit and share the information that underpins their judgements, and involve lay people in the process of decision making. Professionals will only be fully trusted if lay people understand how and why decisions are made and feel that they were involved in the process:

> *Encounters with the representatives of abstract systems, of course, can be regularised and may easily take on characteristics of trustworthiness associated with friendship and intimacy. This may be the case, for example with a doctor, dentist or travel agent dealt with regularly over a period of years. However, many encounters with the representatives of abstract systems are more periodic or transitory than this. Irregular encounters are probably those in which the evidential criteria of reliability have to be especially carefully laid out and protected, although such criteria are also displayed in the whole range of lay-professional encounters.* (Giddens, 1990: 85).

Thus, the nature of professional decision making is clearly central to the effective management of risk through the development of trust. In the remainder of this book we will explore how and in what ways this trust relationship can be developed.

COMMENT

In both traditional and modern societies individuals experience threats to their personal well-being and therefore need and seek ways of creating and sustaining personal security. The anxiety and fear created by insecurity is harmful, especially if it is experienced in the crucial early stages of personal development, childhood. In traditional society, individuals use personalised systems as the basis of their personal security. They seek security from their localised kin networks or from local experts who they know by reputation. In modern society individuals can also call on immediate and short-term support from localised personal networks of immediate family and friends. However, the security provided by these networks is limited as they are usually unable to deal with major threats such as a life-threatening illness. In such circumstances, an individual requires high levels of resources and considerable expertise. Furthermore, these local networks are highly variable. Some individuals develop and sustain extensive networks, whereas others are virtually isolated. In particular, vulnerable individuals such as individuals with learning disabilities or very elderly people are unlikely to have the resources to sustain extensive networks. Thus, in modern society, local networks need to be supplemented by the 'safety net' of health and welfare services which should provide security in a crisis and for particularly vulnerable individuals. Thus, in modern society, the greater the vulnerability and threat, the more the individual has to rely on and trust services provided by professionals such as nurses. In a crisis, individuals often have to trust strangers.

The key issue which the individual nurse has to address is how he or she can develop a relationship of trust with the individual who uses his or her services, especially when they may have no previous knowledge of or relationship with that person. In the remainder of this book, using the concept of risk, we examine ways in which a trust relationship can be developed and sustained. At this stage we will only make some preliminary comments.

The development of a relationship of trust depends on an individual user's general perceptions and experience of nursing and their specific knowledge and understanding of a nurse. If they have no knowledge of a specific nurse then their general perceptions will be of paramount importance, whereas if they have a well-established relationship then this may be more important than their general perceptions. For example, a regular user of mental health services may distrust mental health nurses in general but trust his or her own nurse.

General perceptions of nursing are likely to be heavily influenced by ways in which nurses are trained and the ways in which their practice is monitored and controlled. The very existence of the UKCC and the national boards which set the framework for professional education and practice is designed to provide reassurance to the public in general and the users of services in particular. Of particular importance is the code of conduct which the UKCC publishes and which should provide the framework for the relationship between nurse and patient. The *Code of Professional Conduct* (UKCC, 1992) establishes the standards and framework for professional practice.

However, the actual significance of the code of conduct will depend on the ways in which it is used. If individual nurses are unaware of the code of conduct and disregard it, then it will be brought into disrepute; in other words, there will be a reduction in the level of trust.

Codes of ethics are generalised and impersonal – in Giddens' terms 'abstract systems' (Giddens, 1991). As we have argued, trust is very much about the concrete and personal aspects of relationships. It is embedded in the personal relations between a nurse and patient, and through it the 'personalized front for an impersonal system' (Gilbert, 1998: 1014), individual users judge it in terms of their personal experiences. Thus, if the nurse is to gain and sustain the confidence of the patient or user, he or she has to create the right impression by looking and acting the part and fulfilling expectations (Gilbert, 1998: 1014–15). Clearly one of these expectations is that the nurse can provide the user with security. This will depend on the individual nurse's ability to assess the nature of the threat to the individual and provide ways of counteracting this threat.

The way in which this is done will have an impact on the nature of the relationship. The user needs to be convinced not only that the nurse has the appropriate expertise and can mobilise the appropriate resources but can also use this knowledge and resources in a way which enables the user to reestablish and/or maintain control. Thus the decision making has to be both transparent and shared, ensuring openness and empowerment.

In the next chapter we explore whether current approaches to assessing and managing risk tend towards user empowerment or towards professional domination.

Risk: empowerment or control?

Andy Alaszewski   Helen Alaszewski

INTRODUCTION

This chapter explores the ways in which nurses and other professionals define risk and the implications which these definitions have for their roles and clinical practice. In particular, it will identify three definitions and models of nursing.

◆ risk as hazard and the nurse as a hazard manager;
◆ risk as dilemma and the nurse as a risk and dilemma manager;
◆ and risk as risk taking and the role of nurse as empowerering risk taking.

The discussion will lead into an analysis of the concept of risk and alternative approaches to risk such as risk analysis, risk perception and risk management.

NURSES, VULNERABLE INDIVIDUALS AND RISK

Risk management is now acknowledged to be an important part of professional practice in general and nursing practice in particular. The UKCC has recently adopted a 'risk oriented' mission statement:

Protecting the public through professional standards   *The UKCC is the regulatory body for nursing, midwifery and health visiting. Our purpose is to establish and improve standards of nursing, midwifery and health visiting care in order to protect the public.* (UKCC, 1999: 2)

Within the original UKCC (1992) code of professional conduct, risk is implicit. However, recent elaborations of the code specifically identify the importance of risk. For example, the *Guidelines for Mental Health and Learning Disability Nursing* published in 1998 included a section on risk management and discussed its importance in the following way:

Risk management   *The risk management process should enable the optimum level of care to be given to a client. Risk management involves the assessment of risk relating to client care, care systems and the environment of care. The calculation of risk must be based on your knowledge, skills and competence and you are accountable for your actions and omissions. You should value the process of risk taking, following assessment and in the context of appropriate management, as it will increase your ability to help clients to achieve their potential. However, you should be aware that there may be conflicts between your professional accountability and the autonomy of the client. Although it is rarely possible to eliminate risk entirely, you are still responsible for attempting to reduce risk to an agreed acceptable level. This level should be agreed within the inter-disciplinary team and, where possible, with the client.* (UKCC, 1998: 22).

Mental health

The growth in interest and concern about the risks of caring for and supporting vulnerable people in the community has been particularly evident for people with severe mental illness. There is a major concern about the dangerousness of people with severe mental illness both in terms of self-harm and harm to others. Concerns about self-harm have focussed on high rates of suicide and the Department of Health is committed to reducing these suicide rates. One of the Department's 'Health of the Nation' targets was to reduce the overall suicide rate by at least 15% by the year 2000 and the suicide rate of severely mentally ill people by at least 33% by the year 2000 (Department of Health, 1997a).

Concerns about harm to others have been prompted by a number of high-profile incidents in which psychiatric patients have killed others. The official inquiries into these incidents have identified the importance of risk assessment as a mechanism of identifying and controlling dangerous individuals. For example, the inquiry into Christopher Clunis's murder of Jonathan Zito at a London underground station in 1992 highlighted the key role of mental health practitioners as risk assessors (Ritchie Report, 1994) and the report of the Confidential Inquiry (National Confidential Inquiry, 1999) confirmed their role in ensuring the provision of safer services.

There are parallels between mental health nursing and child protection social work. Although the intention of the child abuse inquiry panels was not to seek individual scapegoats, nevertheless 'there can be little doubt that discovering who was to blame dominated many of the panels' thinking' (Reder *et al.*, 1993: 135). The York study of competencies in mental health nursing also identified a major concern with risk assessment in its survey and linked it to high-profile incidents within the field in the following way:

> *In the wake of recent violent incidents involving people with mental health problems ... attention was drawn to the responsibilities of nurses in relation to risk perception, assessment and management. Whilst there is a sense in which nurses have always assessed risk, and been charged with the responsibility of communicating concepts of risk to clients, practitioners are increasingly being required to adopt a systematic approach to the assessment and management of risks to and from clients. It is axiomatic that the underpinning knowledge and skills must be addressed in preregistration education.* (Lankshear *et al.*, 1996: 173).

The failure of services to effectively manage risk has been so serious that it has called into question the whole commitment to caring for vulnerable people in the community. For example, on the 17 January 1998, the *Daily Telegraph* announced that 'Care in the Community is Scrapped' (Thomson and Sylvester, 1998), and cited a report that one murder was committed every 2 weeks by individuals who have a history of mental illness and about 1000 commit suicide each year. The editorial entitled 'Care before Community' summarised one view of the current state of official policy:

> *A sad and sorry episode in the history of British social theory is drawing to a close. The policy known as care in the community, which plucked the mentally ill out of huge Victorian asylums and sent them to live, often alone, in towns and villages, is to be reversed. Instead, as Frank Dobson, the Secretary of State for Health, reveals in this newspaper, they will be placed in small, secure care homes.*
>
> *The fashionable, sociological solution was to place people with 'personality disorders' in the community, where they would, it was argued, be able to maximise their potential. To suggest that they might be better off staying in secure accommodation was seen as the worst kind of condescension.*
>
> *The experiment went wrong from the beginning. All too often, there was no care and minimal community. Vulnerable individuals, a high proportion of whom had no experience of living on their own, were cast adrift. Their*

families, when they played a role, were often placed under impossible strain.
Many of the former psychiatric patients were dependent on regular
medication. Left to their own devices, they stopped taking it and their
behaviour became erratic. Some committed suicide, others murdered
innocent people. Many of the rest ended up in prisons, hospitals or sleeping
on the streets. The police, prison staff and charity workers tried to cope but
often had neither the training nor the resources. (Daily Telegraph, 1998: 25).

There is little evidence to substantiate the view that ex-psychiatric patients
are a particular danger to strangers and that the development of community
care has resulted in increased danger (see, for example, Scott, 1998: 306). As
Clare Jeffrey of Mental Health Media, an organisation which aims to improve
relations between the media and mental health service users, noted:

the Audit Commission shows that homicides by people using psychiatric
services have slightly decreased since care in the community began ....
Department of Health research also shows that a person is 13 times more
likely to be murdered by a stranger who is 'normal' than by someone using
psychiatric services. (Jeffrey, 1998: 21).

However, public perceptions of risk are not based on objective statistical
information. Bizarre events and actions, especially those which result in significant harm to innocent victims, attract media attention so that rather than
being recognised as exceptional, they are seen as normal or typical. The
media coverage tends to amplify certain risks and has been associated with
exaggerated fears of certain types of hazards. As Scott pointed out:

The media, in the UK, often discuss deaths associated with mental health
problems in a sensationalist and stigmatising manner, with headlines such
as 'Freed to kill in the community' (Daily Express, 2/07/93) and 'Mistakes
let psycopaths kill' (Daily Telegraph, 30/04/96). (Scott, 1998: 306).

This type of distortion has been referred to as 'moral panic', when the source
of fear is a specific group within society (see Cohen, 1972), but is also evident
in 'food panics' such as 'listeria hysteria' (see for example, Kitzinger, 1999).
Thus, whether they like it or not, nurses providing support and care for individuals with severe mental illness in the community have to be aware of public anxieties and the expectations that they will protect the public by
managing risk effectively. Indeed, ministers seek to reassure the public that
nurses and other professionals will ensure that there is no risk:

The Conservative Health Ministers pledged, when announcing the proposed
Patients Charter: Mental Health Services ... that patients would not be sent
home if there was the 'slightest risk to carers, relatives or the public' ....
(normal type shows emphasis in the original, Scott, 1998: 306–7).

Learning disability

In the development of services for people with a learning disability, the concern with risk has come from a different source – from concerns about the ways in which people with learning disabilities were harmed by the process of social exclusion. To counteract this, there has been an emphasis on ordinary living. Thus, while the debate within the field of mental health has tended to focus around the best way to assess dangerousness and prevent the harm that severely mentally ill individuals might cause to themselves or others, the debate within learning disabilities has tended to focus on the best ways of providing people with learning disabilities with the opportunity to take 'reasonable' risks. Perske made this point in the following way:

> *Many who work with the handicapped, impaired, disadvantaged, and aged tend to be overzealous in their attempts to 'protect', 'comfort', 'keep safe', 'take care', and 'watch' ... they will overprotect and emotionally smother the intended beneficiary. In fact, such overprotection endangers the client's human dignity, and tends to keep him from experiencing the risk-taking of ordinary life which is necessary for normal human growth and development.* (Perske, 1972: 195; see also, Wolfensberger, 1972: 203–5 and Saunders, 1999: 64).

This approach was influenced by the Jay Committee, which reviewed services for people with learning disabilities. The Committee addressed the issue of risk in its discussion of the development of alternative care for children:

> *The question of risk, which at this stage involves such things as climbing and running, and later in life hazards of other kinds, is one of extreme delicacy for those who care. Staff are likely to receive harsh criticism when accidents or injury occurs, yet if we entirely cushion people against these dangers we immediately restrict their lives and their chances of development. This restriction can be cloaked in respectability and defended on the grounds of protecting mentally handicapped people and keeping them safe, but it can also endanger human dignity. Each of us lives in a world which is not always safe, secure and predictable; mentally handicapped people too need to assume a fair and prudent share of risk. As we explain in para 308 each unit should have a well defined policy on risk taking.* (Jay Committee, 1979: para. 121).

The Jay Committee recognised that ordinary living and the associated risk taking raised significant issues for vulnerable individuals, between risk taking and protection. The Committee outlined a clear process for risk management. Each unit should have a risk policy which provided a framework for decision making:

Residential care staff will have to implement multi-disciplinary decisions about how far mentally handicapped people can be allowed to act independently, with all that that implies in terms of risk. We have already indicated that we do not want mentally handicapped people to be completely insulated from the day-to-day risks to which everybody else is exposed, but the balance between acceptable risk taking and irresponsibility on the part of residential care staff is a delicate one which varies from case to case. Guidance about risk taking should be included in the Unit's operational policy but the Unit Head will have to take individual decisions after consultation with his own staff, other professional advisers and parents and relatives. (Jay Committee, 1979: para. 308).

Twenty years after the publication of the Report of the Jay Committee, the Social Services Inspectorate (SSI) reviewed the development of the services for adults with learning disabilities. The SSI accepted the basic principles established by the Jay Committee – that adults with learning disabilities had a right to normal life experiences – and it stressed the importance of effective risk assessment in ensuring that such rights could be safely exercised:

The principles also laid the basis for addressing issues of autonomy and of risk in policy and practice for seeking life-styles and activities for users to bring them more into the mainstream of society. Such activities could range from getting the bus to the day centre rather than a door-to-door taxi, and working in potentially hazardous environments, such as kitchens, to having a boy or girlfriend or raising children. (Fruin, 1998: para. 6.5).

However the SSI could find little evidence that service agencies had developed effective risk strategies. It appears that practice falls short of the ideal. As the SSI noted in its report:

In some cases, although staff may have undertaken a risk assessment prior to supporting people in new activities, case files did not record these assessments and decisions. Within SSDs (Social Services Departments), we found it difficult to determine a consistent line to risk-taking issues, particularly where these were not well documented. Even where they existed, not all staff, nor users and carers, were aware of written guidelines on risk-taking. (Fruin, 1998: para. 6.6).

The failure of agencies to develop and their employees to implement effective risk management policies can be linked to a number of accidents and to relatives' and carers' lack of trust and confidence in them.

There have also been high-profile incidents involving people with learning disabilities, but generally these have been ones in which the individuals themselves have been harmed. For example, in 1998 there were two accidents resulting in the deaths of individuals with learning disabilities who were taking part in leisure activities. In September 1998, Barry Denne, an adult with learning disabilities, went missing and was subsequently found dead while on a holiday in Majorca that was organised by a private residential home (the *Guardian*, 1998a: 5). In August 1998, John McGill, Beverly Wilson, Peter Burgess and Eric Jones, all adults with learning disabilities, died in an accident on a canal holiday. The week-long holiday had been organised by the Mill Lane Day Centre in Cumbria. Mike Siegel, Director of Social Services for Cumbria, said that all the staff and users at the centre were devastated by the accident and:

> *Canal trips are a common activity at this Centre and this group has been on holiday together before. Of the four who died, some had attended the Day Centre for the best part of 20 years. They had been active members of the local community, taking part in many of the ordinary community events and involved in education, health and employment schemes in Barrow.* (the *Guardian*, 1998b: 10; see also the *Guardian*, 1998c: 5).

There is some evidence that families do not feel that their vulnerable relative is getting adequate protection. Thus, in the areas of learning disability and mental health, movements have developed which command some support amongst relatives campaigning for more secure and protected facilities. In the case of learning disability this can be seen in the Village Community movement. This movement was closely associated with the Camphill Trust and its origins can be traced back to the immediate post-war era with the establishment of the first village for adults with a learning disability in Botton on the Yorkshire moors. The prime leader of the movement in the UK, Dr Karl König, stressed the importance of developing a secure, safe and, by implication, risk-free environment for vulnerable people:

> *Camphill ... should always grow into a place where those children, not attaining sufficient improvement to go out into the world, could remain and have a useful life .... They should [live] in small houses in the lap of the family to which they belong and where they feel safe and secure.* (Cited in Pietzner, 1990: 50–51).

Older people

Risk has also been a central theme in the care and support of vulnerable older people within the community. The literature concerned with older people recognises both the need to ensure that older people have rights and choice and at the same time that they are vulnerable to and need protection from harm. For example, the SSI's report on older people with mental health problems started its discussion of risk in the following way:

> *Most older people with mental health problems who live alone live at risk –*
> *their choice to live alone makes this inevitable. For them, the benefits gained*
> *from living independently outweigh the risks involved, and the choice is*
> *willingly made.* (Barnes, 1997: 38).

Sometimes these two aspects of risk rest rather uneasily together. For example, a conference organised by Age Concern Scotland around the issue of 'Rights, Risks and Responsibilities' included a paper by a Professor of Philosophy which argued that professionals did not have any right to interfere with older people to protect them from harming themselves (Downie, 1989) alongside a detailed discussion by the Chairman of Age Concern Scotland about falls in older age (Williamson, 1989). The tension between empowerment and protection are clearly exemplified by the conference chairman's introduction:

> *The theme Age Concern Scotland has chosen to highlight this year is that*
> *of falls in old age. A not inconsiderable problem …. The … treatment for*
> *injury sustained and the implications for consequent pattern of living and*
> *human misery are immense. Today's subjects are inevitably part of that*
> *scene as of many others. Rights of the individual and of the professionals*
> *to take risks and carry responsibilities are inextricably intertwined.*
> (McInnes, 1989: 5).

The conflicting pressures on nurses working with older people create dilemmas. Whereas mental health nurses are under strong pressure to prevent harm to the public and client and learning disability nurses have developed a strong client-empowerment philosophy, nurses working with older people find themselves in an intermediate position. They are under pressure to prevent harm to vulnerable clients from the activities of everyday living, such as falls, and at the same time are being encouraged to enhance the independence and autonomy of older people. These tensions are clearly identified in the Sheffield study of the educational preparation of nurses to provide care and support for older people. They noted in this area of nursing, 'the dilemma of balancing safety/risk with a person's autonomy and independence' (Brooker *et al.*, 1997: 134), and commented that:

> *Universally high scores in relation to the promotion of patient safety suggest*
> *that nurses may find it difficult to determine an appropriate degree of risk*
> *and may unwittingly be threatening the personal autonomy of older*
> *patients and clients as a consequence.* (Brooker *et al.*, 1997: 182).

Safety and empowerment form two distinctive strands of research and writing on care of older people that tend to pass each other by: one strand focusses on risk assessment, seeking to identify the factors which predict that an older person is 'at risk' of harm from accidents and other hazards and therefore requires special support; the other strand focusses on 'risk management' and is more empowerment-oriented, seeking to counteract 'ageism' by stressing the positive aspects of risk taking.

The risk assessment approach is very much concerned with identifying the causes of accidents and preventing them occurring. This approach is well exemplified by a study undertaken by the Age Concern Institute of Gerontology to develop the findings of a DTI study (Department of Trade and Industry, 1990) that:

> *Older people are one of the groups of the population most vulnerable*
> *to accidents, particularly in and around the home.* (Wright with Whyley,
> 1994: 3).

The research involved interviews with frail older people, relatives of people with dementia, district nurses, local authority and private agency home care organisers and assistants who were asked, inter alia, 'about their personal experience of domestic accidents and the safety hazards they perceived for older people at home' (Wright with Whyley, 1994: 26). They found that gas appliances, electric appliances and, especially, falls were major hazards and described the significance of falls:

> *Inevitably falls were the most common type of accident described. Three*
> *common underlying reasons appeared to be ill health, excessive alcohol*
> *consumption, and environmental factors. In addition, a significant number*
> *of falls appeared to be spontaneous, with no obvious underlying cause.*
> (Wright with Whyley, 1994: 27).

The significance of falls as a major threat to the welfare of older people was described by Gibson (1990: 296):

> *Falls are the most frequent and serious home accident involving the elderly.*
> *Everyone involved with older people is familiar with their fear of falling*
> *and of the serious consequences which may result from a fall .... Older*
> *people's fears of suffering a serious injury from a fall are real. In the United*
> *States, there are 172,000 hip fractures per year among persons aged 65 and*
> *older. The incidence of hip fractures increases steeply after age 50, and is*
> *highest among the very elderly. Among those who live to 90 years of age,*
> *32 per cent of women and 17 per cent of men will suffer a hip fracture ....*
> *Falls among the elderly carry high societal as well as individual costs*
> *because they result in heavy demands on both short-stay and long-term*

health care. In the US, it has been estimated that the economic cost of all hip fractures is in the neighbourhood of $7 billion per year.

In the UK, the significance of falls has been recognised by the Department of Health (1997a):

More than half of the people aged 65+ who die from accidents die from the effect of falls .... In 1993/94, over 60,000 people aged 65+ were admitted to hospital because of hip fracture, 80% of whom were women.

One of the Department's 'Health of the Nation' targets was to reduce the death rate from accidents among people aged 65 and over by at least 33% by the year 2005.

The other strand of work which emphasises risk management highlights the restrictive nature of services and especially their tendency to exaggerate the vulnerability of older people, therefore restricting them unnecessarily. The starting point for this approach tends to be ageism, or the stereotyping of older people as incompetent and dependent, which needs to be challenged through strategies which enhance the independence and autonomy of older people (see, for example, Bytheway, 1995). This approach was clear in the final report of a project commissioned and published by the English National Board:

Through discussion with the Board commissioners [of the research], it became apparent that the research needed to examine the extent to which programmes of nurse education could challenge stereotypes of ageing. A focus upon the dual concepts of autonomy and independence provides a mechanism for exploring nursing education's challenge to ageism. According to Butler ageism is a process of systematic stereotyping of people on the basis of age. Wade suggests that such stereotyping allows younger people to see older people as different: 'thus they subtly cease to identify with their elders as human beings'. (Brooker *et al.*, 1997: 8, normal type shows emphasis in the original).

It was also evident in a recent review of risk and older people in residential care:

Risks are sometimes taken in order to develop skills and knowledge. This is particularly important for an older person. Many ageist assumptions are made about this stage of life – people often forget that older adulthood is a period of development. Older people need to develop skills to manage the changes (which could be many) in their life. However, it must be remembered that risk taking can sometimes involve losses as well as gains. (Pritchard, 1997: 81, normal type shows emphasis in the original).

It is clear that risk has become an important feature within all aspects of nursing practice. In the early 1990s risk was implicit within codes and guidelines produced by the body responsible for the regulation of nursing, the UKCC. It was covered under the general requirements that nurses should ensure safety and should foster user independence. By the end of the 1990s, risk had become explicit; for example, it was explicitly discussed within the guidelines for mental health nurses.

Risk is also evident in discussions about the best ways of supporting vulnerable individuals within the community. However, the emphasis within these debates is different. Within the area of mental health, there have been a number of high-profile incidents in which individuals have harmed themselves or others. There is little evidence that people who are mentally ill present a particular danger to people they do not know. Indeed, the confidential inquiry into suicide and homicides noted that:

> *Any public health strategy for preventing suicide would have to focus on alcohol and drugs at least as much as on mental illness.* (National Confidential Inquiry, 1999: 8).

However, these isolated incidents have been the source of media interest and government action. The government has put into place measures designed to ensure that the risk which individuals with mental illness pose to others is assessed and, if necessary, managed.

Within the area of learning disability, the emphasis has been on harm caused by the social exclusion of individuals with learning disabilities in isolated institutions. Thus, the main concern has been to provide such individuals with the learning experiences provided by ordinary living and the associated risks. However, such an approach has its tensions. Occasionally things go tragically wrong and there are accidents in which individuals with learning disabilities are seriously harmed, even killed. Furthermore, there may be disagreements between nurses, other professionals and families about what actually constitutes a serious risk, with families having a more cautious, risk-averse or safety orientation. This tension can be seen in support amongst some families for more protected environments, even a move back to institutions – although these are now called village communities rather than hospitals.

Within the field of human ageing, there have been two parallel debates. There has been a debate about the vulnerability of older people, especially to accidents such as falls. Within this debate the main concern has been to assess and prevent risk. The parallel debate has been about sustaining the autonomy and independence of older people and therefore providing opportunity for reasonable risk taking. There has been some awareness of the tension between the two approaches and the need to develop a balanced approach; i.e. one that balances the risk of accidents against the autonomy provided by reasonable risk taking.

THE IMPORTANCE OF RISK IN NURSING PRACTICE

In our study, we invited nurses to comment on the importance of risk in nursing practice. There was strong agreement that risk was an important part of contemporary nursing practice. Of the 72 interviews, there was only one interview with a group of ward nurses in which the respondents did not initially agree, although even this group did eventually agree it was important.

Respondents felt that risk permeated all aspects of nursing practice and decision making.

A lecturer for a post-registration degree course in mental health emphasised the importance of risk assessment for the delivery of appropriate nursing care:

Interviewer: Do you think risk is an important part of practice?
Lecturer: Well, yes, it must be. Very – it seems strange to say this when on the one hand people seem to be saying that risk assessment is an area which has been neglected, it's fundamental and basic. If you don't assess risk properly and get it right you might be delivering totally inappropriate care and it all might go horribly wrong.

Another lecturer for the adult branch of a registration diploma course discussed the importance of risk in terms of the hazards of everyday nursing practice:

Nurses are taking risks all the time. It (nursing) is about calculated risk ... knowing when you can take the risk within your competence – knowing when it's an extension of your knowledge and skills – knowing when it's outside your knowledge and skills. It's knowing what you don't know.

A practising mental health nurse emphasised the way in which risk permeated all aspects of practice:

Interviewer: Do you think risk is an important part of practice?
Nurse: Yes ... it's really I suppose to an extent the risk is, it runs through every ... every aspect of practice and ... you know as I was saying there is always the consequences ....

For nursing students, especially those who were nearing the end of their training and preparing to take on the full responsibility of a qualified practitioner, awareness of risk was linked to their concerns and anxieties about taking on full professional accountability. Thus, they tended to emphasise consequences for nurses if they failed to assess and manage risk effectively. One student described this in the following way:

the weight of responsibility falls on the nurse these days – you carry the can if anything goes wrong.

This concern with safety and accountability can also be seen in the following extract from an interview with a qualified mental health nurse who was undertaking a further post-registration course:

Interviewer: How important do you think risk assessment and management is in professional practice?

Nurse: Oh it's very important in practice you're protecting or to try to prevent accidents happening or anybody getting injured, as a professional person it is your duty, your responsibility to make sure that everybody's safe without any kind of injuries or accidents or incidents while they are on duty or visiting, that's the way I look at it.

There was a clear view amongst the nurses we interviewed that assessing and managing risk formed a central element of nursing practice and a key element of the nursing role. They all agreed that a competent nurse had to have the skills to effectively assess and manage risk.

DEFINING RISK

Most of the nurses in our study treated risk as something which was self-evident. When we asked them how they defined it most of them did not have a ready-made answer. They had to pause to think about the question. Indeed, some of them were initially reluctant to offer a definition.

When they had organised their thoughts about risk, they tended to adopt one of two approaches. The overwhelming majority of nurses (66, 92%) saw risk in terms of the consequences of actions or decisions. One student on the adult branch of a registration course provided the following definition of risk:

You assess the danger and you've got to take certain risks in nursing. If you've got a patient, you weigh up whether it's going to be advantageous to the client or whether it's going to end up a risk. It's when you've done something even though it might have adverse consequences, e.g. smoking, health promotion.

A substantial minority (35, 49%) emphasised the chance or probability aspect of risk. A general nurse who was undertaking a district nurse conversion course emphasised the probabilistic aspect in terms of uncertainty:

It's a thought, an intuition, a judgement about something. A risk is when you're not 100% sure of it.

There was an overlap between the two approaches, with a minority of nurses (29, 42%) including both chance and probability in their definition. Two general nurses who were undertaking a district nurse conversion course linked probability and consequences in the following way:

Student A: ... A risk is when you're not 100% sure of it.
Student B: There's an element of potential danger – ending up in court.

Thus, the nurses in our study tended to see risk in terms of the outcomes of actions or decisions and some nurses also linked this to the probability of such an outcome. In the remainder of this section, we explore variations in approaches to risk.

Risk as hazard

Although most nurses saw risk in terms of outcomes of actions or decisions, they primarily saw it in terms of the negative outcomes of such actions or decisions. These nurses tended to see risk in terms of the cause of such outcomes; in terms of hazards that caused harm. For example, a qualified mental health nurse who mentored nurses on a registration mental health degree commented:

I see risk as a very negative thing because most of the risk that I'm dealing with is the risk of people self-harming or committing suicide ...

A student on the learning disability branch of a registration degree also used a negative image:

Somewhere I used to work – I took a client to the supermarket and he completely smashed the place up and there were children hanging around. It could have been a risk.

Nurses who saw risk in terms of the harmful consequences of hazards used negative images, often emotionally charged or multiple images, to emphasise their point. One mental health nurse referred to the Dunblane incident in which a socially isolated man shot schoolchildren, their teachers and then himself, while in another interview a district nurse made the point by repeated examples:

Risk can be ... it's when there may be a problem of harm; basically something going wrong; everything has a risk attached to it so it could be risk of injury to the patient, risk of injury to the staff; in organisations there is risk which they have to look at with people coming into the buildings.

There's risk of injury through spillage; making sure your equipment's safe that you are using; you haven't got harmful substances lying around; things are locked up; keeping the risk of harm to a minimum.

Risk taking

A minority of nurses stressed a more positive aspect of risk. Although they acknowledged the possibility of things going wrong they focussed on the process rather than the outcome, stressing the positive aspects of the process of risk taking. They saw risk taking as a learning or therapeutic process that was beneficial for the users of services and used a more positive definition. A lecturer on a learning disability course defined risk in the following way:

Well, risk is a very important area in learning disability and anybody working in that area needs to be concerned with it. It is enabling the people you work with to do something, but taking into account the risk that may be involved ... for example, you might have somebody who is suffering from epilepsy and you may want them to take part in a certain activity – you need to make a judgement about what the risk to that person is and that's got to be balanced with the experience that they get by taking part, so it's taking account of the risk involved without devaluing the person by not letting them take part.

Nurses with this approach tended to argue that risk was not an objective fact, a hazard that could be identified with the right technical expertise; rather, they adopted a 'social construction' approach, seeing risk as a social category that could change according to the social and power relations. They implied that many 'risks' were artificial. Excuses were used to restrict opportunities for service users. For example, in response to the question: 'What do you understand by risk', one learning disability nurse commented:

Very interesting question. In the learning disabilities field we talk a lot about risk because ... clients have not taken risks or not been allowed to take risks due to the nature of care that we provide. And it can be anything from something very small like putting the kettle on, which was often regarded as a high risk for several people, to being left in a house on their own ... it's entirely down to the individual as to what you would class a risk as being; something that's a risk to you or I may not be a risk to somebody else. (It) depends on your own abilities, your own perception and also the person with learning disabilities – their perception of what a risk would be.

Nurses using this approach also employed emotional imagery but they drew their images from positively valued social activities. A qualified nurse who mentored the learning disability students used an image of a dangerous but valued activity, bungee jumping. A nursing lecturer on a learning disabilities course used another example of a leisure activity to illustrate her response:

A real life example is ... a girl I worked with some years ago who was quite able and made friends with some men in a pub and two of them invited her to a party and she really wanted to go. It was like no, but in the end she did because she's got a right to go. But it was like thinking it through. [It was] not a case of what I allowed her to do but ... what has she let herself in for basically.

Risk as a balance of consequences

Approximately half of the respondents acknowledged both the positive and negative aspects of risk and therefore saw risk as a balancing process in which probability was of crucial importance. Thus, if taking a risk could have a harmful consequence while not taking it would be a missed opportunity, the issue of choice and the probability of different outcomes was of central significance. A qualified learning disability nurse identified the importance of the process of decision making and of balancing positive and negative outcomes:

Interviewer: What about enabling clients to make decisions. Is that an aspect of practice you'd associate with risk?

Mentor: Balancing ... [clients] don't have insight into all the areas that you're talking about and would choose to go off when they've got no road safety skills. You know that's their choice but with a duty of care you'd have to balance that with what the risk was and your responsibility to ensure that they were (safe).

Respondents developed relatively complex images to illustrate the process of balancing positive and negative outcome. They used images of everyday activities, such as cooking a meal, smoking a cigarette or walking across a room, but associated them with dramatic images of harmful outcomes, such as fires and falls which were a product of the vulnerability of the clients. A mentor for students on the adult branch of a registration degree course first emphasised the vulnerability of a client, then drew attention to the harm the patient had experienced and finally noted the everyday activities which had resulted in this harm – smoking and drinking cups of tea:

We had a gentleman when we were on our previous ward who had a degenerative disease affecting his coordination and was in quite an unbalanced stage; his potential for self-harm at that stage was huge really, his movements were very, very erratic ... he did get hurt on several occasions – he was a smoker and there was a potential risk there that he was going to injure himself with cigarettes, which made it difficult, and hot cups of tea things like that; obviously we'd try and cool them down as we could but a cold cup of tea is nothing compared to hot cup of tea.

Students on a learning disability registration ENB course identified the everyday activity but left the potential harm implicit:

Student A: It's like when you're teaching somebody how to be independent and take a bus themselves ...
Student B: Or crossing the road.
Student A: ... when do you actually leave that person to get on that bus themselves say and meet them at the other end or whatever; those kinds of risk came to my mind which ...
Student B: Particularly road safety; I was thinking of that.
Student C: Yes, a service user learning to cross the road for instance.

It is clear that the dominant definition of risk amongst the nurses in our study was the everyday definition of risk as hazard or danger and as something to be avoided. However, we also found other views of risk. A minority of nurses saw risk in terms of the positive process of risk taking, which is valued in its own right as it provides individuals with excitement and status. More prominent was the view of risk as a balance between positive and negative outcomes. In the next section we explore the extent to which the definitions can be identified in different areas of community nursing.

VARIATIONS IN DEFINITIONS AND ASSOCIATED ROLE PERCEPTIONS

We included within our study nurses from three main specialisms: community nurses, nursing disability nurses and mental health nurses. For all three groups the dominant or primary approach to risk was in terms of hazard and danger. Thus, risk was seen as a threat that had to be countered. In all areas it was possible to identify alternative approaches: either risk as an opportunity or risk as a balance between positive and negative outcomes. It was most difficult to identify these subsidiary approaches within mental health nursing. Risk as *balance* was mostly clearly articulated amongst nurses caring for older people and risk as *opportunity* was most clearly developed within learning disability nursing. The differences were even more marked when we considered the examples which nurses gave to illustrate their definitions. Of the

28 images used by mental health nurses, 17 (61%) related to the serious consequences that could result from clients' behaviour, such as violence, suicide or fire. Of the 27 images used by nurses specialising in care of older people, 18 (67%) related to the harmful consequences of everyday living, such as falls, pressure sores or hypothermia. Of the 39 images used by learning disability nurses, 24 related to the activities of daily living such as crossing the road and catching a bus.

Mental health nurses

Mental health nurses tended to see risk as a threat, especially the threat posed by clients' actions: either self-harm such as suicide; and for dangerous clients, harm to others – especially the public – such as violence. An experienced community mental health nurse defined risk:

> *What do I understand by risk? ... the big thing is whether or not the people we are working with are going to remain alive or not ... the biggest area of risk is around suicide, para-suicide, be that deliberate or accidental, so that's the area that's very much at the sharp end; there's issues around risk of self-neglect and vulnerability as well. Again I think there was a classic case about a year or two ago ... where two users of the mental health service who also had drug and alcohol problems, one killed the other, he split his head in half with an axe ... there are a lot of dangerous people out there ... in one year I saw three people who were referred to me for stress management who had all served prison sentences for arson ...*

Respondents were concerned that their practice was increasingly influenced by high-profile incidents in which acutely ill people had harmed themselves, members of the public or staff and which had been the subject of public inquiries and media attention:

> *if you're talking about somebody who's actually talking about committing suicide, then yes, choice is certainly a factor in terms of how you might work with them ... making decisions to take their choice away ... all the reports on people like Christopher Clunis and others, where there are lots of evidence [that] this guy was likely to be a risk to others and to himself. Was he given any choice or did we, did we take it seriously?*

A qualified mental health nurse working in a secure unit described the impact of the media in the following way:

> *The Unit has received a bad press. You only have to open the papers. I think this morning there was a sex offender escape from a medium secure unit ....*
> *As soon as anything like that happens, it has a knock-on effect for client*

decisions that are made about the client group. It depends politically what happens.

Respondents using this definition of risk tended to see the prime role of the nurse as a manager of the hazards associated with providing care and support. Thus, their main role in relation to risk was to identify the hazards and to minimise harm to clients and others.

Again, this approach dominated in mental health, and respondents emphasised the role of the nurse as an identifier and manager of hazardous client behaviours, especially self-harm and attempted suicides. An experienced community mental health nurse described his role as a hazard manager in the following way:

> *There's issues around risk for me as a practitioner, around whether or not I am physically safe to practice or whether I'm professionally safe to practice. If I get the decision wrong how does that affect me and my profession and my organisation? The physical side again is something that will broadly focus with me. I got a 'good kicking' when I was on call 6 months ago; that's happened. It's happened twice in the last 15 years. It does happen and it can happen.*

There was in this approach a concern to identify 'risk factors' and to develop objective and scientific measurements of them:

Researcher: What about safety. Is that something you would associate with risk?

Nurse: Yes, mainly around the self-harm and harm to other people; but I think, again as a manager, being aware of legislation around health and safety at work, COSHH regulations, manual handling, those kind of things, and heightening staff awareness around those kinds of issues – infection control. We're having to get quite involved in both infection control and manual handling now.

Learning disability nurses

In our interviews with learning disability nurses, risk as a threat was also prominent but they also discussed risk in terms of opportunity. Nurses who challenged the dominant approach tended to argue that risk was not an objective category and therefore there was no agreed checklist of hazards: each individual and each situation was unique, and hazards should not be used as an excuse for preventing reasonable risk taking. A qualified learning disability nurse not only emphasised the subjective aspect of risk but also linked it to a personal experience of thrilling risk taking:

Interviewer. What do you understand by risk?

Mentor. That's a really difficult question to answer; it depends ...
Who's defining it? What might be a risk for me might be
totally different for somebody else. I've just been white
water rafting OK, and I did not assess the risk before I
went; if I'd done my homework and watched the videos
before I undertook this then I might have felt very
differently but I got swept away on this sort of notion that
this was the thing to do whilst one was on holiday. But I
was in the position of being able to make that decision and
I was taking the responsibility for that decision even
though I hadn't assessed it properly .... And that's very
different from somebody who's receiving a service and is
dependent; I'm reluctant to use that word dependent – I
suppose who is having other people sum up or assess what
the risks are ...

Thus, respondents using this approach to risk felt that they had to challenge
'common-sense' approaches which individuals built up through their pre-
nursing experiences. These were defined as 'prejudices' that needed to be
countered, as in the following extract from an interview with a lecturer on the
learning disability branch of a diploma registration course:

> *It is multi-dimensional – one person's risk is not another's. Risk is to do
> with perceptions based on one's past experiences. It's a very difficult concept
> to teach students because they have to be aware of their own feeling and
> prejudices. For example, with the risk of allowing consenting adults with a
> learning disability to have a homosexual relationship, I try to help students
> come to terms with the problem of defining risk.*

Nurses using this approach were often self-consciously reacting against the
traditional institutional or hospital care in which patients were 'cocooned'
in a supposedly safe and secure environment. They argued that the benefits
for the residents were illusory. Deprivation of the stimulus of everyday life
and risk taking was associated with stereotypical behaviours designed to
provide self-stimulation such as rocking or masturbation. In practice the
institutions 'protected' the public by removing and isolating people
with learning disabilities. Respondents who adopted this approach to risk
tended to see the nurse's role as primarily an enabler who facilitated risk
taking by individuals. An example which was often used to illustrate this
approach was enabling a person with a learning disability to undertake an
activity of everyday living which might be dangerous, such as making a cup
of tea:

Researcher:	What do you understand by risk?
Student A:	The chance of some negative consequence happening.
Student B:	Giving someone the opportunity to do something which might have harmful consequences: making cups of tea; running baths; using hot and cold water; crossing the road; promoting independence.

Nurses using this approach had to use their judgement about what was a reasonable risk. They tended to see this as a judgement based on their special knowledge of the skills and ability of each client. Thus, nurses had to use their judgement to decide how and when to teach a service user to cross a road. In this approach, decision making was seen very much as a shared process with the client identifying what activities he or she would like to undertake and the nurse assessing how and in what ways they could facilitate the activities. The service user and nurse needed to develop a shared understanding and responsibility for increasing the client's range of activities and risk taking. A student nurse on a learning disability degree course gave the following example:

> *I work with someone, and there was a huge risk meeting to decide whether this person was allowed to go to the post office on his own or not. It was decided that he could. He had the sense and the knowledge to be able to cross the road and to get the money and sort all that out. But what no-one had taken into consideration, until after the event, was the time when he went to the post office to get his money and two guys in a car stopped him and asked him if he wanted to go the seaside; he got into the car, but somehow managed [to provide a diversion]. I think he said: 'I haven't got enough money or I need my tablets,' or something, so they drove him to the house where he lived, and at that point the car was intercepted and stopped. But the scenario hadn't been thought about previous to that and now he won't go out without anybody because of that incident.*

Nurses caring for older people

Nurses working with older people in the community are aware of the possibility of accidents, especially falls, but most want to balance these against positive objectives, such as maintaining the older person's autonomy and independence. A student nurse on a post-registration course specialising in the care of older people commented:

> *You can assess risk and the care someone is going to get from you allowing them to take that risk. I'm thinking particularly of a lady who regularly had falls on our ward but who didn't like the restriction of movement – that made her very unhappy and quite agitated – which she felt it was*

impinging on her privacy and independence. After discussion we decided, with her and her family, that she would sooner take the risk of having the falls and breaking a bone, or whatever, rather than have somebody following her round, as that impinged on other things which she thought were more important to her. I think sometimes, even if the risk is greater, i.e. that the person may injure themselves, they gain something in other ways at an individual level. Nurses are not 100% sure that a patient will get a pressure sore but they're not prepared to take that risk.

Nurses working within this framework tended to see risk in terms of dilemmas: the difficulty of making choices when there were high levels of uncertainty or conflicts of interests and values. For example, a qualified nurse working on a ward for older people identified the dilemmas associated with providing care for an elderly patient with a serious degenerative disease and, in particular, the tension between protection and empowerment of a patient:

His potential for self-harm at that stage was huge really; his movements were very, very erratic; he could still mobilise, but he was as likely to bounce off the walls as he was to actually walk in a straight line, and it was very difficult to see that happen; but we came to a decision that there was no way we could try and restrict his movements at all – he ... had all the rights that we possess as well. We could quite easily have restricted his movements by putting him in a room with very little furniture in it, maybe a mattress on the floor, but that wouldn't have been right, so we decided that we would take the risk and allowed him to do these things: we'd take the risk if he was going to get hurt .... It's very difficult, because as a nurse you want to care, you want nurture, you want to look after people and protect them from the ill-effects of treatments that we might give them whilst also advocating treatments we know may help – that was difficult.

Nurses who recognised the dilemmas of caring for vulnerable individuals identified several strategies for resolving these dilemmas. These included exercising their own professional judgement to make a choice or using their ability to negotiate agreements which reconciled conflicting interests or objectives. For example, in their discussion of issues raised in relation to protecting the public, students on the adult branch of a diploma registration course identified the dilemmas created by conflicts of interests and the need to use value judgements to resolve them:

Student A: Well, come to think of it, maybe driving, as well you know; if someone has had two TIAs [transient ischaemic attacks], maybe you should be informing the driving, you know DVLA [Driver and Vehicle Licensing Agency] and stuff, yeah, I suppose again, it's not something we've (covered in the course).

Student B: Yes, it's a lot of value judgement ... circumstances that aren't covered by legislation ....

Student A: The thing is that they ... to begin with you're taught not to be judgmental and not to bring your own feelings into it.

Student C: Yes, values and beliefs.

Interviewer: Into it, yes, it's hard.

Student C: As time, as time goes on they're the only things that you're sure about ... your judgement or lack of it or your beliefs, because you're weighing up something against them to decide if it's right or if it's wrong .... I mean there's no way that you cannot be judgmental about some things.

An alternative approach to the same dilemma was to adopt the stance of an independent arbiter and seek to negotiate an agreed solution. A lecturer on a district nursing course commented that:

Part of allowing people to stay at home. If you've got older people living on their own it's that balance – it's the danger to themselves and the danger to the neighbour – it's when you start looking and say how far down the line can I go with these risks. But if someone is adamant, that they do not wish to move, in many ways it allows them to take that risk. If I was a client I would want to feel that my students were pulling out all the stops to allow me to take that risk.

COMMENT

All the nurses in our study recognised the importance of risk for their professional practice. However, they did see risk in different ways. Most saw risk in terms of the consequences of actions or decisions: especially harmful consequences and outcomes. Thus, the dominant view of risk was as a hazard or danger to be avoided. There was less emphasis on the positive aspects of risk, especially the potential benefits to be gained from risk taking and little on the probabilistic elements of risk, that implied an evaluation of the probability of different types of outcome. Risk as hazard was prominent in all aspects of nursing, and was particularly evident in mental health nursing. Risk as a balance of probability could also be identified amongst nurses specialising in care of older people, while amongst learning disability nurses it was possible to identify risk as an opportunity for reasonable risk taking which could benefit users.

Service users, informal carers and risk

Jill Manthorpe   Andy Alaszewski

INTRODUCTION

In Chapter 2 we explored nurses' perceptions of the importance and nature of risk. We showed that nurses saw risk as an important part of practice and that they tended to define it in terms of hazard and their role as hazard managers. In this chapter we explore the ways in which other stakeholders, especially users and informal carers, view risk. If there is a systematic difference between nurses' and other perceptions of risk, then it is important that this tension is identified and resolved, otherwise it will undermine the partnership between users, carers and nurses.

USERS, CARERS AND RISK: SOME STEREOTYPES

In the UK, the pattern of services for vulnerable people has shifted from long-term care within institutions towards care and support within the community, if possible within the vulnerable person's own home. Underlying this shift is a consensus amongst politicians, civil servants and professionals that institutional care is both expensive and harmful. Underlying this consensus is a downward 'risk escalator' (Heyman and Henriksen, 1998: 96–103) in which a partnership between user, professionals and informal carers increases the skills and social integration of the vulnerable person, thus progressively reducing the risk to which they are exposed and the level of therapeutic interventions needed to manage these risks. Scott described this approach for people with mental health problems:

> *rehabilitation programmes preparing patients to return from psychiatric hospital to the community were devised as sequences of small steps which, when successfully accomplished, would give the individual, their family, and the public, confidence in their ability to live with greater freedom and autonomy. Such positive reinforcement was expected to lead to the increasing integration of patients into the 'community', and, in turn, to reduced levels of patients stress and the consequent risk of relapse. In this virtuous circle, individuals would progress to the point at which they could live with little or no support from mental health services.* (Scott, 1998: 307).

This process depends on mutual trust and confidence between users, carers and professionals. This trust is likely to be undermined if users, carers and professionals do not see risk in the same way. One of the main tensions within community care has arisen because it is claimed that participants have different approaches to risk and that the dominant professional approach is not shared by carers. SANE, a major mental health pressure group, captured this tension in the slogan it used to attack current professional practice:

> He thinks he's Jesus. You think he's a killer. They think he's fine. (SANE, 1989; poster cited in Scott, 1998: 303).

In other words 'he', the service user, is too ill to be aware of risk; 'they', mental health professionals, fail to recognise the risk and take appropriate action to protect the user and others; while 'you', the lay person, with your 'common sense', can clearly identify the risk but are likely to experience the harmful effects of professional misjudgements.

Scott argued that a reading of official inquiry reports into incidents where individuals with severe mental health problems have caused serious harm tends to provide support for such stereotypes. In a minority of these reports there was evidence of professionals consistently ignoring families' concerns about dangerousness:

> *Professional views often stand in sharp contrast to those of both the public and families of people with schizophrenia. Inquiry reports show that professionals repeatedly minimised the significance of violent incidents .... Official reports contain numerous examples of desperate but unanswered appeals from parents and other close relatives, friends and voluntary workers.* (Scott, 1998: 309).

In the literature on learning disabilities, similar stereotypical views can be identified. As Corkish and Heyman (1998) pointed out, the literature on family care of adults with learning disabilities depicts carers as responding to their vulnerability by stressing the dangers and hazards that may be associated with risk, portraying:

> *adults as restricted by their care environment, and family carers have been represented as trying to maintain their offspring in a childlike state.* (Corkish and Heyman 1998: 216).

Professionals, by contrast, are said to stress the importance of risk taking and the opportunity which it offers social and personal development, strenuously advocating their clients' right to take risks. In this they drew on a well-established literature which, as Heyman *et al.* (1998) wrote, placed a positive value on risk taking:

> *The academic literature on the lives of people with learning difficulties strongly favors risk. Perske ... refers to* 'the dignity of risk' *for the mentally retarded. The notion of parental* 'overprotection' *(Block) incorporates a covert value judgement that parents ought to encourage people with learning difficulties to take more risks. The concept of* 'letting go' *(Richardson and Ritchie) implies that parents avoid risk for adults with learning difficulties for selfish reasons, because they do not want to give up the parental role.* (Normal type shows emphasis in the original; Heyman *et al.*, 1998: 211).

Thus, professionals and support workers often saw family carers as over-protective, emotionally dependent upon adults or financially motivated to keep their charges in a state of pseudo-childhood (Heyman and Huckle, 1993: 1562). Family carers, however, sometimes felt that professionals and support workers pushed for change and urged them into dangerous situations because they lacked intimate knowledge of the adult's limitations. Nevertheless, most professionals interviewed by Heyman and Huckle (1993) believed that these adults with learning disabilities failed to achieve their real potential.

Since the 1960s, there have been a growing number of accounts in which people with learning disabilities speak out for themselves (see Atkinson and Williams, 1990: 6–7). These accounts consistently demonstrate a desire to undertake some of the riskier activities of adult life. For example, in *Peterborough Voices*, Eve commented:

> *Why am I rebellious? I don't know, to tell you the truth. It was probably because at school I used to be a goodie, goodie, so I wanted to change my role a bit, and I knew damn well I would get a clipped ear from my Mum*

and Dad. But because Mum and Dad weren't around I knew I could do what I wanted. (Peterborough, 1997: 7).

While Enzo described his marriage in the following way:

My parents thought I'd stay at home all the time. Basically they didn't want me to move away from home. On the other hand, I've got my own life to lead now. I still go and see them when I can. I've always been close to Mum and Dad and my sister. And that will never change. I think they find the change very difficult. Mum and Dad feel they have lost me but they haven't .... They've always been very protective .... They overreact too much. They overprotect so much. (Peterborough, 1997: 13).

In one of the few studies of the attitudes of family carers and adults with learning disabilities towards risk in purely community-based environments, Heyman and Huckle (1993: 1557–64) found that most adults with learning disabilities and family carers overtly saw risk in the same way. However, differences did occur and usually resulted in direct conflict. Family carers tended to assume that they could be aware of all their relatives' needs without consulting them and, more significantly, without feeling any obligation to do so. Difficulties generally arose when adults expressed needs that family carers did not perceive. Heyman and Huckle commented that such behavior might fulfil a psychological function for family carers: 'ignoring' some potentially risky desires of adults might enable them to minimise some of the perceived losses to the adults they support arising from danger avoidance (Heyman and Huckle, 1993: 1560). There also appeared to be a concerted effort made by family carers to (over)compensate for this by engaging the adult in activities requiring carer involvement.

Heyman and Huckle (1993: 1560) found that adults with learning disabilities and their family carers used evidence from their own experience to maintain or shift their classification of hazards as risks or dangers. Such evidence often took the form of 'horror stories' used to reassure carers and their charges that imposed limits were necessary. However, these tales often related to the adults' childhoods, with little allowance made for their changing circumstances over the years.

Family carers tended only to permit those activities which might have been considered 'normal' for a young child within a family. Relatives are said to see the adults with learning disabilities that they support as irresponsible because they fail to appreciate the consequences of their actions and desires. Family carers consequently respond to this perceived irresponsibility by stressing the dangers and hazards that may be associated with risk, regarding their relative as a perpetual child incapable of balanced decision making. Thus, adults' risk-taking behavior was clearly confined within a controlling family environment (Heyman and Huckle, 1993: 1561). Overt conflict between adults and family carers arose when adults systematically rejected the limits imposed by their families by seeking the freedom to engage in activities such as independent living, work, sex, marriage and parenting (Heyman and Huckle, 1993: 1561).

In the area of human ageing, stereotypes can also be identified but the pattern is a bit different. Rather than being irresponsible, older people are often stereotyped as intrinsically cautious and risk averse. The ageing process is seen as making them more conservative. This can be seen particularly in regard to crime where older people's subjective 'fear' of crime is not justified by the 'objective' crime level. The role of the professional is to realign subjective 'fear' and objective reality either by education to reduce the fear level or by introducing safety devices that reduce objective risk. Reed (1998) described the stereotype of older people's response to crime in the following way:

> *Their [older people's] responses to crime can seriously affect the life quality of older people (Cook et al.). Hough and Mayhew among others, have argued that older people overestimate the threat of violent attack or robbery, since, statistically, they are less likely to experience such crime than younger people. This literature portrays older people as living defensively, and dismisses their fears as irrational. Suggested remedies include, as so often, educating them about 'real' risks, and encouraging them to use security devices. The literature thus appears ambivalent as to whether older people's fears are to be changed by education, or reduced through security precautions.* (Reed, 1998: 248).

Reed suggested that this 'professional' approach to risk underpins most of the discussions of the ways in which older people see and respond to risk:

> *Much of the material concerned with risks for older people is produced by professionals, researchers and policy-makers, and reflects their perspectives. Images of frailty and vulnerability predominate. Responses to these images express either paternalistic concern with protection, or an equally paternalistic promotion of risk-taking. Both positions fail to take into account the ability of older people to make their own decisions.* (Reed, 1998: 251).

The situation of mentally competent older people differs from that of adults with learning disabilities and individuals with severe mental illness, as there appears to be relatively limited attention to the risk perceptions of a key third party, the informal carers or family. However, in the case of mentally incompetent older people, for example individuals suffering from dementia, this third party becomes important and the focus of interest shifts from the older person–professional relationship to the carer–professional relationship. In Clarke and Heyman's 1998 review of the literature on risk management of older people with dementia, this shift is so complete that the older person – professional relationship is not even considered. In this literature the older person with dementia does not have an input or voice, thus by implication lacks any responsibility for assessing and managing risk.

Clarke and Heyman presented and analysed stereotypes of the carer – professional relationship and these differ from the stereotypes in other areas. They argued that carers used social models of the situation and emphasised their own personal knowledge of the older person and the unique personal identity of the person who has dementia:

> *In order to protect this individual knowledge base, and to find the evidence to support it, family carers seek out exceptions to the professionally defined, pathological, view of dementia. They do not necessarily deny the inevitability of deterioration, but use any signs of intact personhood in their relative as evidence that they are still the human being known in the past.* (Clarke and Heyman, 1998: 230–1).

Carers used risk-taking strategies to sustain their definition of the situation of 'normal' life for as long as possible. These strategies may involve explicitly challenging professionals by rejecting their services as:

> *Acceptance of any professional carer intervention entailed the implicit or explicit admission that there was 'something wrong' with the person with dementia, and could increase the interpersonal distance between the 'normal' family carer and the 'not quite normal' person with dementia.* (Clarke and Heyman, 1998: 236–7).

Clarke and Heyman argued that professionals operate within a medical or clinical perspective which emphasises the abnormality of the situation and the need for professional intervention to protect the older person. Professionals see the carers as unrealistic, irrational and failing to realistically evaluate risks, so creating a potentially dangerous situation. This is not a view that Clarke and Heyman share:

> *Professionals often see client non-compliance with their risk-management recommendations as irrational: as rash or overprotective. Family carers, such as Mrs G, discussed in the opening example, who insisted that her mother should sleep upstairs despite the risks involved in getting her downstairs, and Mrs Y, who allowed her father to wander rather than have him put on medication, are very much 'risk experts', with their own distinct forms of contextualised risk knowledge and reasoning. They actively manage risks, on the basis of this knowledge, through the process of interfacing.* (Clarke and Heyman, 1998: 240).

Despite the limited research on the ways in which service users and informal carers define and respond to risk, this has not prevented commentators from both describing and prescribing how various stakeholders respond to risk. Given the absence of empirical data and the tension underlying much of the debate, it is hardly surprising that stereotypes abound. Perhaps the most common stereotypes are of users being irresponsible, as they are not able to fully appreciate the nature of hazards; informal carers as risk averse and excessively cautious, tending to exaggerate both the vulnerability of users and the threat posed by hazards; while professionals encourage user to take risks, minimising threats. As we pointed out, in some areas the pattern of these stereotypes can be different; for example, in caring for older people with dementia, the informal carers may play the role of optimistic risk takers while the professionals are pessimistic and risk averse. Clearly it is important to be aware of the difference between definitions of risk because, as Clarke and Heyman pointed out, they may be a major source of tension and conflict:

> *Bradbury ... argues that science-based approaches to risk presume the superiority of expert over lay knowledge. Professionals who uncritically take for granted their epistemological superiority may seek to educate family carers, through a one-way communication process, about the risks they face, and to promote compliance with their advice. However, the effective management of health problems requires mutual client and professional understanding of each other's risk knowledge. Otherwise, professionals will not value family carers' knowledge, and family carers will dismiss professionals' advice as inappropriate.* (Clarke and Heyman, 1998: 239).

Stereotypes can be a useful starting point for research; indeed in the social sciences they have played an important role as 'ideal types'. However, they may conceal as much as they reveal and in the next section we draw on our research to explore the usefulness of these particular stereotypes.

BEYOND STEREOTYPES: TALKING TO USERS AND CARERS

When we interviewed service users and informal carers about risk we did not find clear stereotypical responses. As with our interviews with nurses, there were variations in opinions and views. Indeed, there were strong similarities between our group interviews with nurses and those with service users and informal carers. It was clear that all groups saw risk as an important issue but they also treated it as a 'taken-for-granted' idea so they did not have ready-made answers. Individuals needed to pause to think about it and in some cases wanted prompts. However, once they got into the flow, most groups had a great deal to say about risk and how it affected their lives.

Similarity of views

Within these discussions it was possible to identify similar debates about the nature of risk and similar themes could be identified. For example, one of the themes identified in our interviews with nurses was risk, and especially risk taking as a normal part of everyday life. The three quotes in Box 3.1 are all drawn from individuals involved in learning disability services.

Extract A is taken from a group interview with informal carers; Extract B comes from an interview with a learning disability nurse; and Extract C comes from an interview with users of learning disability services. Although there are clues in each extract about the identity of the speaker, the actual definitions of risk are virtually interchangeable; for example, Extract C from the service user is both clear and confident.

Another prominent theme within nurses' interviews was risk as danger and the harmful consequences of failing to identify and deal with hazards. We demonstrated how amongst nurses caring for older people this was particularly associated with falls. The three quotes in Box 3.2 are all drawn from individuals involved in services for older people.

Box 3.1 Individuals involved in learning disability services

Extract A: Well I think living life is a risk, so it doesn't really enter my mind.

Extract B: There has to be an element of risk in everybody's lives, walking across the road's a risk ... Life is one big risk. Clients have to take risks.

Extract C: It's a chance – like taking a caravan on the M25. Take risks on the road and crossing it. You look and listen before crossing.

Box 3.2 Individuals involved in services for older people

Extract D:

A: If you lose your balance or something ... because if you fall you're on the floor and that's it, you probably can't get up you see.

B: I think falling is the worse.

C: Yes, you know if you lose your balance for any reason I think that is the worse.

Box 3.2 Cont'd

B:	You fall in the bath don't you.
C:	Well, yes, anything, I mean if you're down you're down aren't you.
A:	Yes, that's right, you can't get up at all.

Extract E:

Question:	What do you understand by risk?
Answer:	By risk? I suppose it's anything where somebody is in any kind of danger. It's very broad really with the sort of people that we deal with; I mean we're aware of and involved to a degree in risks at home and in the community ... the most common areas perhaps are physical problems – people falling at risk, at risk of falling, wandering – and as far as possible we try and eliminate those risks.

Extract F:

I fell out of the back door one day and I thought 'my goodness that could have been it' ... you wouldn't believe what went through my mind just as I fell out that back door ... I thought, 'well I could be laid up and what's going to happen to Bess?'

Again there are clues within these extracts as to the identity of the speakers. Extract D is from an interview with older service users, Extract E is from an interview with a nurse specialising in the care of older people; and Extract F is from an interview with informal carers. However, there are strong similarities between the underlying theme in each interview. In each there is a concern with vulnerability and the serious consequences of failing to identify hazards that could result in a fall.

Shared approaches to risk

Our interviews with service users who had established long-term relationships with services tended to identify the influence of service providers' perspectives on risk. Just as nurses tended to see risk mainly in terms of hazard, most of the participants within our groups also saw risk in terms of hazard, although again we were able to identify 'undercurrents' of conflicting approaches.

Like learning disability nurses working in this area, service users saw risk primarily in terms of negative consequences:

User A: I used to live in an old house and there was a risk of fire because of electrical faults.

User B: When it gets dark it's risk and safety. There is the risk of being abused. If you go out at night – people on skate boards – you get abused if you don't get out of the way.

One group of service users we interviewed had a very limited understanding of risk and spoke purely in terms of dangerousness, things that might hurt them or which might be 'too hard'. They responded to a prompt about bungee jumping in the following way:

Interviewer: What if you wanted to do something new, like bungee jumping, on a big bit of elastic? Would the staff here help you to do that?
Mark: They'd say too dangerous ...
Janet: No, they'd say no.
David: Oh, I don't know ...
Interviewer: Would they say it's too dangerous?
Janet: Yes.
Mark: It's too hard, too hard isn't it.
Janet: Might fall off ...

The participants were mainly concerned about the impact of these hazards on their lives. They clearly felt that these hazards prevented them developing full lives and contributed to their social exclusion:

Jean: If I say something they take no notice. At the college I wanted to put my name down for a Christmas dinner and they made it so I couldn't. They shouldn't have done that. That's the risk of college – being ignored .... I've been stopped from going somewhere. I should be able to go, to do what I wanted to do. They said I shouldn't go – you won't know about it.
Simon: Our group organised a disco. Most people lived in the city – it was in the city – but people wouldn't go because it was in the city on a Friday night and they said it wouldn't be safe.
Tom: And my holiday. I was going to Spain but the staff said they were having difficulties getting some people able to go. The travel firm was seeing people in wheelchairs as a risk.
Jean: We're not taken seriously.

The users discussed the strategies which they had developed to deal with hazards:

Simon: If it's wet – should I take a risk of walking along the pavement? I watch how other people walk and copy them.
Tom: If cars are coming I wait for the lights to change.
Simon: There are the basic rules which can take away some of the risk.

It was possible to identify in the interviews with users of learning disability services a theme which was also evident in interviews with learning disability nurses: risk as a form of empowerment, so that successfully taking risk is a positive experience. One service user described this in the following way:

> *I went to [major seaside landmark] – there was a sand dune – it was hard to get up – we went up. We took pictures. It was a risky thing but worth it. Someone was with us.*

Within our discussion with users we could find little evidence to support a stereotype of individuals with a learning disability as unaware of risk and therefore irresponsible. Indeed, they were acutely aware of the hazards of everyday life and the impact on their lives. Not only were most participants in our groups keen to show they were responsible, identifying hazards and learning to manage, but one user took this a step further. She demonstrated her responsibility by helping a less-able user take risks:

> *I go with Joseph to a [large supermarket] because he doesn't understand roads and can't understand money. He throws money away. If he had a £10 note he would just give it away.*

Like mental health nurses, users of mental health services saw risk as hazard. One group of service users consisting of people with enduring mental health problems, including manic-depression, depression and anxiety, had clearly discussed the issue of risk before. Our question about risk provoked a lively discussion in which it was possible to identify some of the examples used by professionals, such as suicide:

User A: Are we a risk to the public? It's always put in the paper – if there's a murder, it blows up if it's schizophrenia. If it's a normal person it's OK.

User B: Risk – like are they [professionals] qualified to make sure they're the right tablets? We don't like being doped up. Medication is risky if we don't get the right one.

User C: There's the risk of being sent back to work – a risk of relapse.

User D: Risk – well it's about suicide. I'm considered a high suicide risk. When I'm high with my manic depression, I'm very wary of missing a doctor's appointment. I've used the phrase 'I'm a high risk suicide'.

This excerpt demonstrates a variety of understandings of risk. The users were clearly aware of the narrow hazard-oriented definition current both in professional and media discussions of mental illness. However, they also identified the hazards associated with the treatment of mental illness, such as the side-effects from medication: in other words, they noted that some treatments can have negative or unintended outcomes as well as beneficial results. The expert role of those professionals prescribing medication was questioned.

In our interview with the users of mental health services we developed the discussion by inviting the group to consider the impact of risk on respondents' everyday lives. A prominent concern was the management of medication and associated relations with professionals. One user identified risk in two aspects: the interaction of his medication and alcohol and regularity of consumption. He managed his medication by adhering to a strict routine. Another respondent stated that she managed to remember her medication by following a set routine but also knew that if she missed an appointment she would be contacted by phone. A third user referred to his problems in remembering medication and his fixing of set times. As a safety net he knew that if he missed an appointment with his key worker, a nurse would call on him within 24 hours:

> *I know they'd [professionals] do it because they would worry. There's a bush telegraph in mental health. If the warning signs start, they know.*

This interview demonstrated both the similarity and differences between professional and users' perspectives. They shared a common concern with harm, for instance suicide, and also a common understanding of the way it could be managed for people with enduring mental health problems, such as taking medication and meeting regularly with professionals. However, there was a difference in perception of control over the situation. Nurses saw themselves as structuring the relationship, while users clearly saw themselves as playing an active role, especially in managing their own risks. Users had a variety of strategies for managing their situation, which included:

◆ using professionals such as nurses as a safety net;
◆ helping to manage exceptional situations;
◆ and reducing the likelihood of high levels of negative consequence occurring, for example, suicide, self-harm, acute illness episodes.

Older service users were also aware of the hazardous and precarious nature of their situation. Like nurses working in this area they were well aware of the risks of their everyday life, and showed similar concerns to professionals about the ever-present possibility of accidents such as falls. For example, in one user group the first and immediate response to the question about risk was falls:

Interviewer: What does it [risk] bring immediately to mind if we mention that word?
User A: The risk of falling.
User B: Yes.

Like nurses, older people were aware of the hazards presented by their homes and the harm that could result from an accident. Thus, their own home rather than being a safe environment was potentially hazardous. For example, they felt they were more likely to have an accident such as a fall inside their home than outside. Another hazardous activity in the home was cooking. For example, one older woman shared a common experience in the kitchen with others:

User A: Well we're crippled most of us and your hands start trembling like; you'll have a plate in your hands, it looks as though it's waving or you have a pan of peas and they finish up on the floor.

User B: Or your dinner.

User C: Or your dinner slides off the plate.

Some users saw risk as all-pervasive and applying to all areas of life. They had to learn to balance the potential negative consequences with the positive aspects of life. One older user commented: 'You take a risk for anything don't you?' and 'we're always at risk'.

Risk involved negative consequences and chance. These older people illustrated their understanding with examples from their own experiences: 'You take a risk when you have an operation don't you?'.

They saw risk as part of their everyday life, as something they had to learn to live with:

Interviewer: And do you think if we talk about risk that it's about things that will happen or things that might happen?

User A: I think it's about things that will happen and again.

User B: Yes they do happen; not probably, they do happen.

User C: You can't say when they are going to happen but it just happens.

As with nurses supporting older people in the community, users were aware that they had to balance the hazards of everyday life with maintaining their independence. One older person described the way she maintained her personal hygiene in the following way:

Doris: I get a bath every day with a board.

Interviewer: Do you get help with that?

Doris: No, no.

Interviewer: You do that on your own.

Doris: Yes, yes. I'm frightened but I do it.

Interviewer: Who provided the board?

Doris: The welfare .... I have a cord [life-line] in every room. Social services [provided it] but I go out every day.

Service users clearly saw risk assessment and management as an important part of their lives and drew on common-sense definitions. Like nurses they tended to use a negative hazard-oriented definition of risk, even when, as in the case of mental health service users, they saw themselves as a hazard to themselves or to others.

Generic carers groups

In our research we identified two distinctive types of carers groups – generic and specialist. The generic groups tended to be groups of carers who were actively involved in caring for an individual at home and therefore they meet for mutual support. The specialist groups tended to be made up of informal carers whose relatives used a specialist facility such as a day centre or a residential unit. The generic groups were often geographically based, bringing together carers in a specific locality; so these carers were providing support for a variety of different vulnerable people. The specialist groups were often linked to a specific facility or service; indeed, their meetings often took place at the facility. We interviewed both types of groups and in this section consider the locality or generic groups.

Like service providers and users, informal carers who were providing continuing care and support for a vulnerable person tended to see risk in terms of negative consequences, as hazard and harm. They did not discuss risk in general terms but related it directly to their personal circumstances and particularly to the vulnerability of the person they were caring for. The environment outside the home was seen as particularly dangerous. For example, one carer discussed risk in relation to her daughter who had learning disabilities:

> *Well my daughter is at risk if she tries to walk and people expect her to walk because she looks quite normal; but if they expect her to walk then she's likely to fall, so she's at risk whenever she's out of my sight really.*

Indeed, many carers saw the external environment as so dangerous that they took measures to ensure that the vulnerable person stayed in the house. Such strategies could themselves be risky, as one carer pointed out:

> *She's at risk all the time so I've taken the key out of the door. This could be a real problem if we need to get her out quickly.*

Since many vulnerable people did not go out independently, carers' concerns were mainly with hazards in the home. Another carer talked about her elderly mother's vulnerability in her own home: 'Thing with mum always falling, she wouldn't use her frame.'

For carers, the vulnerability of the person they were caring for created specific hazards that had to be counteracted through the everyday process of caring. For example, one woman caring for her elderly husband made the point that her husband's loss of sight was central to the risks created in the household:

> *My husband's blind so you can imagine what the risk is there – you know fire and all sorts of electrical things, material things; like we got rid of a gas fire because of the risk and replaced it with an electrical fire.*

These carers had to manage risk effectively. Failure to do so could have disastrous consequences. A carer whose wife was suffering from dementia but wished to carry on cooking described a 'near-miss' in the following way: 'It was 7 o'clock in the morning and all the gas rings were turned on full. The house was full of gas.'

Risk was a part of everyday life and involved not only the vulnerability of and hazards created by the person being cared for but the hazards created by professionals. Carers accepted the support of professionals who worked with them and supported their strategy for managing risk. For example, one carer had fitted a personal alarm system to her mother's bungalow and was pleased that when her mother set the alarm off both the ambulance service and the GP had responded quickly. However, the initial response of one carers' group to risk was to equate the hazards created by professionals alongside other hazards:

Interviewer.	If I said the word risk what would you associate with it?
Carer A:	Do you mean that we think we're at risk by them (professionals) coming into the house?
Carer B:	Do you mean danger?
Carer C:	Fire?

Carers were concerned about professionals undermining their risk strategies. One carer described the disorienting effect of professionals in the following way:

> *Social services; she [my mother] had 46 people careering through her house in a week. They stressed her and took over her home. I had to keep explaining to her, they can be good but they do come in and take over.*

Indeed, some carers found the services offered so disruptive and threatening that they preferred to do without them and manage on their own. One carer said that her husband did not want to be left with a stranger, while another commented:

> *You don't get any choice. They offered us a sitter for 2 hours. We had never met her before; my mother didn't want strangers in her house so we had to cancel the appointment.*

Given the importance of risk in their lives and the strategies which they had developed to manage risk, most carers were worried about their own vulnerability. They felt that they could cope as long as they did not become ill or have an accident:

Carer. I think you worry as well about it, if you become ill ...
Other carers: Yes, yes.

After discussion of a number of other 'risky' activities (for example, standing on stools) this group discussed how they countered their own personal vulnerability. One carer commented that, 'It makes you more cautious.' Some carers restricted their activities as a precaution; for example, two members of the group indicated that they avoided going out as much as possible. This theme was reflected in another group interview, where a number of carers referred to risk in relation to their own health. One man caring for his elderly wife commented:

I worry about my own health .... There is a problem when I have to go to hospital for a check-up .... If my health dives, she'll have to go into a Home.

Another carer referred to the difficulties of sleeping in relation to the uncertainty of looking after someone who he felt could die overnight at any time. Since he slept upstairs and his wife slept downstairs he commented that, 'Every morning I wait for a phone call. [I] open the door and stand to hear.' He linked 'risk' to the physical work of caring: 'It's just constant, we do it because we love them. Physical risk, pushing mum, pushing wheelchair.'

Risk forms an important part of carers' everyday lives. It permeates their relationships not only with the individual they care for but also with others involved in providing care. Like professionals and users they saw risk primarily in terms of hazard and harm. The 'outside' world was a major threat and a source of anxiety, especially if the person they cared for went out independently. However, given the vulnerability of the person they cared for, the home could also be a hazardous environment and carers faced challenges in maintaining a 'safe' home environment.

Carers focussed on risk within their own lives. They tended to see themselves as the major and sometimes sole support for vulnerable individuals, their relatives, and were concerned to develop strategies that enabled them to continue in this role. Although professionals could be seen as a threat to this continued relationship the major threat came from the recipient of care themselves, either through their vulnerability or in some cases as a source of danger. Carers felt they had developed strategies for dealing with risk but generally these strategies depended on their own continued well-being and therefore they were concerned with their own vulnerability.

WORKING TOGETHER: COMMUNICATION
AND TRUST

In the previous section, we examined the views of carers who participated in locality groups. The carers in these groups took prime responsibility for providing care, identifying both the importance of risk within their everyday life and their ambiguous attitude to professionals. In this section we develop our argument by considering the situation of informal carers who participated in groups associated with a specialist service, such as a day centre or residential unit. For these carers, their relationship with their relatives remains important but is now linked to and mediated by the unit and agency providing the specialist care. This creates a more complex pattern of relationships and, particularly in the case of residential services, may change the nature of risk management. In this section we explore the insights generated by our discussions with informal carers in this situation.

When we talked to the relatives of adults with learning disabilities we found that risk was clearly an important issue for them. The majority of family carers were extremely concerned about vulnerability, especially the potential for individuals with learning disabilities to be abused in a variety of ways. As one family carer asserted:

> There's so much abuse happening ... every time you hear the news or open the paper there's that much abuse, physically or sexually or anything.

This vulnerability was particularly evident in major life or fateful decisions. Parents had to address these issues as their child got older and began to move into adult life. One parent identified the difficulty in the following way:

> This is the biggest risk I think in every parent's life, who is a carer .... When is it the right time to let your child go? It's scary because you don't want to hold them back ....

Most informal carers saw risk in terms of hazard and harm, usually the hazards that existed in the environment. One parent of an adult with Down's syndrome and diabetes illustrated the difficulties created by such a combination of conditions:

> It's happened two or three times when we've let him go out with some friends ... with him being diabetic it's a problem, because people will offer him a cup of tea and put lots of sugar in it and he's ended up in hospital because of that. So these are the risks, because he is a diabetic I have to keep an eye on him 24 hours a day .... If his friends offer him a cup of tea he doesn't think to tell them not to put sugar in. At home we have diabetic drinks, Diet Coke and so on, so he can get a drink whenever he

wants – but that's a bit of a risk because he doesn't realise that other people's drinks have sugar in them.

This example is interesting as it illustrates how easy it is for a risk-avoidance mechanism (providing a ready supply of sugar-free drinks) to lead to additional dangers or risks (the assumption that all drinks are sugar-free), which are then more difficult to control or negotiate.

These informal carers were also aware of the potential hazards of the ordinary domestic environment. Although they did not provide continuing care, there were usually home visits. One carer spoke of the potential dangers to be faced when his son visited him for a holiday:

When you take them home and you're in a normal household environment there are lots of things which are risky – normal things to us, but John for instance, has no sense of danger at all; he wouldn't think twice about switching on our old gas cooker and that sort of thing.

In some cases the informal carers may see the vulnerable person as a source of danger and emphasise the aggression or the strength of their relatives:

You know how it is with handicapped kids .... Sally, you know, she's very, very strong and the risks are very, very strong.

Despite their anxieties about risk, the vast majority of family carers, particularly those connected to day services, incorporated risk into their everyday lives. They accepted that 'reasonable' risk taking could facilitate personal development and independence and many informal carers had developed strategies which involved risk taking that involved trusting the person with learning disability. In some cases, this worked very well:

When Brian retired, we started going out together more, and we had to rush back for Mark coming home from school; well we thought about getting him a key. So we put a key on a piece of elastic and it goes in his pocket. The first few weeks we made sure we were home, just in case, and we hid behind the curtains to see what he'd do. We'd shown him how to open the door and come in .... Now it's alright ... he just comes in, hangs his key up – we know if he's in because his key's hanging up – then he'll go upstairs and watch his TV or a video. He'll sit there quite happy until we come in .... That was a risk, but we had to ... he's 29 years old after all.

This parent alluded to Mark's age and this highlights a tension that many parents felt between their child's status as an adult and as a person with learning disability. A small but vocal minority of parents energetically supported the view of an adult with learning disabilities as a 'perpetual child':

Sarah: And at the end of the day, as I always say they're just children in adults' bodies … well they are, most of them … four year olds in twenty-plus bodies ….

Bill: They'll never grow up; I mean, he loves his mum and he loves Christmas, but it's as a child. Martin expects to see a big pile of toys on the chair when he comes down and he always picks the biggest out first to open and that sort of thing.

This view of adults with a learning disability as 'children in adult's bodies' emphasised their mental incapacity and their inability to effectively assess and manage risk. Some parents gave examples in which things had gone wrong. For example, Stephen's parents had used the same risk strategy as Mark's parents. They gave Stephen a key to get in, but this strategy did not work for them:

We tried a similar thing with Stephen [giving him a key] so he could get in if we weren't there, but it was hopeless .… He got that frustrated that he didn't know what to do … if the door was shut he didn't know what to do; he just stood outside because he couldn't get in. And when we weren't there, well that was a big risk.

Thus, family carers in our study certainly did not like taking unnecessary risks and, as the literature in this area indicates, adults with learning disabilities are often seen as perpetual children. However, it was clear that the behaviour of family carers is more complex than the literature tends to suggest. They would embrace risk-taking activities if these were seen as worthwhile and not detrimental to the safety of their relatives with learning disabilities.

When we talked to informal carers in specialist groups about their relationship with service providers, all the families we interviewed were positive about the support they received from specialist service providers, such as learning disability nurses. However, a significant number of carers had 'horror stories' about the services they had received from other professionals. One family carer gave a vivid illustration of this point:

They are very far behind in hospitals in dealing with the handicapped … they don't understand .… Katie had an in-growing toenail, it was infected .… She saw the registrar and he said, 'Well, we'll put her on the list, it will be eight to ten weeks' .… I was a ward sister .… I was in casualty and I knew that we used to whip them off there and then because I mean, you couldn't expect people to wait that long. So I came out in absolute disgust and I said to the staff nurse, 'Does this chap see private patients?' .… So he had me back in and he eyed me up and down first of all to see if I could afford it .… I said, 'Look, I had this problem with her teeth, Katie was banging her head on the wall with the pain and she has got a high pain threshold, and I'm not prepared to go through that again, let alone Katie' .... He just looked at me and said, 'Well actually it would be morally wrong to take your money; would she let me do it under local anaesthetic in casualty?' I says, 'Yes, if I can go in and hold her, she'll let you do it.' And she was as good as gold and I think he was so ashamed because she just popped up and said, 'Thank you doctor!' and he went and fetched her a cup of coffee himself! But you've got to fight all the time if you want anything doing.

The problems that family and professional carers reported with members of the medical profession give us an insight into what they believed was necessary for a good working relationship to be established and maintained. It appeared that a crucial factor in this was trust, built upon a shared respect and understanding of individuals with learning disabilities and reinforced by a willingness to communicate with all those involved in the care and support of these adults. Professional carers had to demonstrate these behaviours in order to earn and maintain the trust of family carers.

Carers recognised that their assessment of risk could differ from that of service providers. As one concerned mother of an adult attending a day centre said:

Professionals will encourage you to let them move on. But you've brought them up, you've cared for them ... you know their capabilities more than anyone else.

However, this difference was not necessarily a source of conflict. When families trusted service providers they were willing to discount their own fears, accept professional judgement and embrace decisions which involved risk taking, even if they themselves would not normally have engaged in these activities with their relatives. This was particularly true when the risk-taking behaviour involved new challenging physical activities:

When my sister came here they wanted her to go sailing, now she can't even swim ... she doesn't even like water. So I wouldn't have let her go, to be honest, but they were happy to do that.

The families we interviewed all had a high level of confidence in the specialist learning disability services which they and their relatives received:

If I had a lottery win come through then this place could carry on as long as these live, that's the way I look at it .... This place is brilliant.

It's wonderful, to know that somebody else can look after them.

A range of factors contributed to this widespread satisfaction. A small but vocal minority of carers had previously experienced services which they felt had broken their trust by failing them and their relatives. In these cases, family carers were content simply because they believed the current service to be 'better'. Several carers of adults in residential care had 'horror stories' about other facilities. As one family carer told us:

> *We went to two or three places with Amy .... One of the places was the queerest place I've ever been in my life. We took Amy through the door and the first thing we got was two blokes fighting ... there was one of them on the floor and the other one was kicking the crap out of him .... I didn't want to leave her there .... The other place; well while Amy was there she lost three-quarters of her finger. We don't know how she lost it; we got one letter from the people saying that they didn't know how she lost it .... She lost about an inch and a half of her finger and they said she must have bit it off ... it's a great person that could have bitten it off like that, never mind a handicapped person .... We think she lost it in a door or something like that.*

Personal experience or second-hand knowledge of breaches of trust such as this caused a number of family carers to admit that they hoped that they would outlive their relative so that they would always be able to monitor their care and support. As a number of parents in one focus group confessed:

> *Anna:* You can't see into the future and at the moment I think, well, Katie's quite happy but what will happen in the future if anything happens to me? ... To be honest, and I'll say this very openly, I really hope Katie dies before I do, and it isn't because I don't care; it's because I do care enough to think about it. I'd like to think that that was it and I knew what the end would be and that was the end of it. I think we all feel like that.
>
> *George:* I think I would feel the same. I think I would hope that I would outlive her.
>
> *Barbara:* I've said it to people who've looked at me and said, 'Oh no, you can't say that!', but they don't understand .... You love them, don't you, but you're just concerned that when something happens to you, what's going to happen to them and if they died before you then you wouldn't have the same worry.

Family carers were aware of the possibility of incidents and accidents and did not expect their relatives to be kept in a risk-free environment. What they did expect was prompt and comprehensive information if something did go wrong:

> *I mean, they have a very good policy of communication with us so if there are any problems they do ring, they don't just sweep anything under the carpet ... you're not thinking, 'Oh, what's going on behind my back?' all the time or anything.*

This confidence in staff and services is crucial if the best possible care and support for adults with learning disabilities is to be provided. All the family carers we interviewed were prepared to trust professionals and devolve what they saw as their responsibility of care, but only if they could be assured that this would not pose a threat to the safety and happiness of their relatives. Thus, their trust was clearly conditional. Family carers saw their role as one of monitoring the work of professional carers, at all times retaining the right to intervene and, if necessary, withdraw their relatives from a service. As one parent explained:

> *He'll always be our responsibility, no matter where he is – we'll always have an over-riding responsibility for him ... where he is we can defend him and keep an eye on him .... We're quite happy for him to be here ... we know he's in good care.*

The issue of conditional trust is of huge importance to all family carers, particularly those connected to residential services. As one such parent argued:

> *With most of our children not able to speak, you have to have trust, because they couldn't really tell us if there was something wrong; anyway ... we have to believe that what we're told happens to them does happen.*

Most family carers also agreed that the views or behaviour of their relatives was an important factor in developing confidence in a service. As one parent reported:

> *When John was being moved around, trying to find a residential spot for him, we tried three residential homes and, although he can't talk, he can't tell us, he walked out of one and he just wouldn't entertain it and the social worker said, 'Well he's voted with his feet, hasn't he!' Now when we came here, he didn't know this place from another and the first thing he did was settle himself down on the settee and he looked as if he was at home. The atmosphere had obviously got to him.*

It was very important to family carers that their relatives were happy, stimulated and safe when they attended any sort of learning disability service. They wanted them to fulfil their full potential. Many carers considered it their responsibility to monitor their relatives' state and they used this as the major source of evidence when evaluating the suitability of a service:

> *Eric is happy here, I think they must be doing the right things or he wouldn't be happy. I don't feel that I really need to know more than that and I know Eric doesn't. He doesn't care about policies, he doesn't understand that sort of thing .... He just knows that his friends are here and he likes it, he has fun.*

Therefore appearance and intuition are important elements in the process of building trust. If the adults using a learning disability service appear to be thriving, are happy and busy, and there is no evidence of harm, then family carers are prepared to trust professional carers. Relatives did not really want to look 'behind the scenes'. For example, they did not seem interested in the policies that underpinned specialist agencies' actions or procedures and tended to take policies for granted unless something went wrong. None of the family carers we interviewed had any real interest in any of the policies or procedural guidelines that were in place, and their comments about these were often very vague:

Interviewer: Are you aware if this agency has a specific risk policy?

Claire: They do have, don't they. They read it out, yes, they read it out ....

Interviewer: Do you know anything about it at all?

Derek: Well, it was read out a couple of times, it covers all sorts of abuse, physical and financial ....

Claire: But I don't really ....

Interviewer: Do you think you are all aware of how these policies work at all?

Brian: Personally, no.

Trust based on concrete personal knowledge and experience is more important than knowledge of abstract policies:

We have a very close connection with this place .... Over the years they have proved that everything runs smoothly and it's very good ... the way they do anything seems to be along the right lines .... I don't really understand the policies here all the time, but I trust the staff here so I don't really feel that I have to.

Parents were interested in processes when it related to their personal lives. Almost all the family carers in our study were aware of how to make complaints and had a great deal of confidence that these would be taken seriously and dealt with. As one commented:

Well, I think it's part of your role as a parent and a carer to say, 'So, what was it all about, who's to blame, whose fault was it?'

COMMENT: DEVELOPING AND SUSTAINING TRUST

Although stereotypes can be useful as a starting point, reality is usually more complex than the stereotypes imply. We could find little evidence to support stereotypical views of service users as unaware of risk and therefore irresponsible, and service providers as advocating risk taking in the face of rather cautious informal carers. We found that users, carers and providers all saw risk in terms of hazard and were aware of the harmful consequences of failing to properly assess and manage risk.

Users, carers and nurses all had very different and, at times, conflicting ideas about the nature of risk and how it ought to be negotiated on a day-to-day basis. Risk is a highly complex notion and it appears that many of the users and carers tended to view it in concrete terms, to be aware of it as it affected their lives, usually as a problem that had to be dealt with. There was a clear degree of convergence between how family and nurses thought about risk, with most agreeing that it was both inevitable and to be encouraged if any predictable dangers could be eliminated. Thus, most individuals agreed that there was a need to balance opportunities with protection. This agreement was complemented and possibly reinforced by the depth and frequency of communication between family and nurses, which enabled family carers to develop a conditional trust of staff and devolve their perceived responsibility of care. However, family carers insisted upon retaining a monitoring role and reserved the right to influence practice and withdraw their relatives from the service if they felt that this trust was breached.

Family carers indicated that they did not fully understand the policies and procedures of professional carers but were prepared to accept that they were well designed and implemented, providing there was a clear relationship of trust between all parties, service users were happy and came to no apparent harm, and professional carers could explain their actions if challenged. The use of this sort of monitoring makes it essential that service providers are aware of risk and how they manage so that they can justify their decisions; otherwise, there is a danger that the bond of trust between family and nurses will be broken.

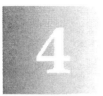

Decision making and risk in individual practice

Helen Alaszewski   Andy Alaszewski

CHAPTER CONTENTS

INTRODUCTION

In this chapter we examine how risk shapes nursing practice in general and decision making in particular. We start by exploring the importance of risk management and decision making in providing nursing care for vulnerable individuals in the community. We then draw on our research to explore how nurses manage risk in their everyday practice through decision making.

PROFESSIONAL PRACTICE, RISK AND DECISION MAKING

We share Dowie's (1999) concerns about the misuse of the term 'risk' and in the early chapters of this book we explored the different ways in which the concept of risk has been defined and used. We noted that nurses and other stakeholders tend to define it in a narrow and technical fashion by concentrating on hazards and the harmful consequences of failures to identify them. Although hazard assessment is important, it is only part of the overall process of risk management and in this chapter we want to explore nurses' overall approach to risk by examining the ways in which they respond to situations and make decisions. We start with a discussion of the literature on risk and decision making in nursing practice.

Risk and decision making

Risk management and decision making can be seen as different ways of referring to the same process. Dowie (1999) argued that we should focus on decisions and decision making rather than risk and risk management, as risk is an ambiguous concept which has frequently been used to disempower people by creating the illusion of certainty and control by 'risk experts'. While Dowie (1999) preferred to concentrate on decision making, his criticisms apply mainly to the narrow hazard approach (and can also be applied to restricted approaches to decision making). In these restricted approaches, the main emphasis is on technical issues – for example, the technology of hazard assessment – and little attention is paid to issues of uncertainty and to underlying value systems.

If we adopt broader approaches to risk and decision making then it is possible to see both the similarities and differences between them. In the sphere of human actions both are concerned with outcomes of actions or choices; however, they emphasise different aspects of the process. Risk refers to the outcome of choices or actions and risk management to efforts to ensure the best outcomes. Decision making focusses more on the process of choice – for example, Dowie defined a decision as a 'choice between available options/strategies/policies' (Dowie, 1999: 46) – but implicit in the process of choosing is an evaluation of the possible outcomes of different choices:

> A decision-making process is defined as the thoughts and actions
> associated with a sequence of choices as well as the choices themselves.
> (Dawson, 1992: 195).

Risk management and decision making need information. Risk management involves the use of information gained from past events to assess the probability of future outcomes. This may be formalised with the use of statistical tools such as Bayes' theorem (see, for example, its application to child abuse by Munro, 1999). Decision making also involves the technical process of collecting and using information to help in the choice process and to reduce uncertainty. Thus, Checkland and Scholes considered information collection as an essential precondition for making a decision. Using Simon's rationalistic approach they identified three elements in decision making:

> Simon's simplification is that managers are decision makers who proceed
> through a three-stage process of intelligence, design, choice. In this first stage
> problems are identified and data are collected; 'design' consists of planning

for possible alternative solutions; 'choice' entails selecting an alternative which is good enough, and monitoring its implementation. (Checkland and Scholes, 1990: 165).

Rationalists see decision making as a technical activity, in which the decision maker should follow a defined sequence of activities to arrive at the best possible decision. Etzioni identified these stages in the following way:

> *Rationalistic models are widely held conceptions about how decisions are and ought to be made. An actor becomes aware of a problem, posits a goal, carefully weighs alternative means, and chooses among them according to his estimate of their respective merit, with reference to the state of affairs he prefers.* (Cited in Smith and May, 1993: 198).

Doubilet and McNeil have also identified three main steps, but their approach established a more explicit link between decision making and risk management. They were concerned with providing guidelines for decision making and argued that decision makers should start with potential choices, then use probability and values as guides to choice:

> 1. *Construct a mathematic model of the decision problem (this is commonly done using a decision tree, which displays the available decision options, or strategies, and possible consequences of each).*
> 2. *Assign probabilities to uncertain events.*
> 3. *Assign values (utilities) to each potential outcome.* (Doubilet and McNeil, 1988: 256).

Thus, risk management and decision making involve value judgements and techniques for coping with uncertainty. However, in both there is also a tendency to simplify the process by concentrating on their technical components. This tends to minimise the complexities generated by value issues and uncertainty. As Green pointed out in her analysis of the growth of the technical expertise of public health specialists in 'accident prevention':

> *In the 'risk society' public health has refocussed its attention on 'injury reduction', and on establishing an evidence base for risk reduction. The accident, with its connotations of randomness and unpredictability disappears.* (Green, 1999: 25).

Dowie in his criticism of 'scientific risk assessment' made the point forcibly, although his comments are equally applicable to 'rational decision making'. He argued that there are two possible interpretations of the misuse of risk:

> *[In the malign/critical interpretation scientific risk assessments] are used knowingly by governments ... to obfuscate, to sustain an exaggerated appearance of control over uncertainty, and to imply that scientific*

> *assessments can lead to policy conclusions – which they cannot unless*
> *combined with value judgements that, by definition, have no 'scientific'*
> *basis .... In the benign (or less malign) form, governments ... are simply*
> *carrying out their function of relieving the population of the burdens of*
> *decision making, taking these burdens up on the basis of an implicit request*
> *equivalent to 'do what you think is best, doctor' .... Talking the language of*
> *'risk' and 'safety' is very much consonant with ... a 'dumb down democracy',*
> *since it enables one to leave outside political discourse all the complexities*
> *of defining and assessing probabilities, of defining and assessing*
> *desirabilities (and aggregating them across individuals), and of articulating*
> *the principle to be used in integration.* (Dowie, 1999: 52).

Some policy makers and civil servants are aware of these issues and want to involve the public in more informed debate. For example, the former Chief Medical Officer of the Department of Health expressed concern about excessive public reaction to 'risk' such as 'food panics'. He argued that the most effective way of preventing such panics was to involve the public in decision making through improved risk communication. In the preface of the book which he edited with a former colleague from the Department they started with the statement that:

> *Decisions about risk are not technical, but value decisions.* (Bennett and
> Calman, 1999: ii).

To avoid the pitfall of 'scientific risk assessment' or narrow expert-based decision making, it is important to address the following three issues.

Reasons why a choice needs to be made

As Doubilet and McNeil (1988: 256) pointed out 'the first step in an analytical approach to clinical decision is precisely defining the problem'. In practice, decision analysis often takes the 'problem definition' for granted (see for example Klein and Pauker, 1988). In risk management, the desired outcome might be taken for granted – for example, harm minimisation – but there may be disputes about the nature of harm. For example, preventing a person with learning disabilities crossing a road may protect them from physical harm but it may expose them to other forms of harm such as social exclusion.

Evaluations, outcomes or consequences

Decision making involves evaluating potential outcomes and making 'an assessment of the un/desirability (utilities, preferences, valuations) for the outcomes' (Dowie, 1999: 46). In rationalistic models of decision making this involves identifying and evaluating all possible outcomes and making choices which maximise utility. Risk management focusses on the benefits of the intended outcome and compares them with potential unintended outcomes.

Assessment of probability or chance

This should be central to both decision making and risk management. Decision makers never possess complete information. Decision making involves making choices in situations of uncertainty and therefore must involve judgements about probability. Narayan and Corcoran-Perry (1997: 354) pointed out that 'decision-making tasks of interest in professional domains are characterised by complexity, ambiguity, and uncertainty.' Dowie and Elstein (1988a: xv) considered that in decision making 'elements of risk and uncertainty are unavoidable, due to the nature of the problems to be dealt with and/or the imperfect character of the knowledge and information available to deal with them.'

In the remainder of this section we focus on risk management and decision making in nursing.

Nursing, risk and decision making

While doctors, especially in hospitals, are generally seen as decision makers, the decision-making role of nurses tends to be less clearly developed and articulated. As Bucknall and Thomas noted in their study of nursing in critical care settings:

> *Nurses were found to be high frequency information providers, but low frequency decision-makers.* (Bucknall and Thomas, 1997: 231).

Perhaps to establish beyond doubt that nurses are indeed decision makers, research in nursing tends to concentrate on describing and analysing the ways in which nurses make decisions.

Analysing decision making

A starting point for an analysis of nurses' decision making is Benner's (1984) widely cited study. Her main interest lay in the ways in which nurses' decision making altered as they acquired experience and confidence and moved from the status of a novice practitioner and decision maker to that of an expert. Benner argued that as nurses acquired more clinical experience, they gained in confidence and the pattern of their decision making reflected this. Newly qualified or novice nurses lacked confidence, so needed external support for their decision making. This support was provided by the rules and procedures which they had learnt during their training. The decision making of these nurses was characterised by the self-conscious use of such rules to justify their decisions:

> *The rule-governed behavior typical of the novice is extremely limited and inflexible.* (Benner, 1984: 21).

In contrast, 'expert' nurses had gained experience and confidence and therefore could dispense with the support provided by self-conscious rule following. Their decision making was more internalised and speedier as they remained confident in their own judgement and in their own ability to grasp the key elements of a situation:

> *The expert performer no longer relies on an analytic principle (rule, guideline, maxim) to connect her or his understanding of the situation to an appropriate action. The expert nurse, with an enormous background of experience, now has an intuitive grasp of each situation and zeroes in on the accurate region of the problem without wasteful consideration of a large range of unfruitful, alternative diagnoses and solutions.* (Benner, 1984: 31–2).

Benner argued that the intuitive decision making which was the hallmark of the 'expert' nurse was more effective for managing risk than the laborious rule-based approach of 'novice' nurses. Expert nurses possessed sufficient confidence and expertise to challenge 'unsafe' decisions made by other practitioners, especially less experienced junior doctors:

> *Nurses are often caught in the ambiguous role of serving as a back-up system to ensure safe medical and nursing care; often this entails altering the treatment plans of other care providers. Expert nurses are aware of the possible avenues for circumventing problems as they arise; they work with a healthy skepticism and ongoing questioning of treatment plans; and they are well aware of their capability to provide back-up safety and to change treatment plans as the patient's condition dictates.* (Benner, 1984: 139).

Offerdy (1998) examined the ways in which nurses working within general practice in England make decisions. Her research explored the extent to which these practice nurses used formalised systems to make decisions. She found that they seemed to be mainly using internalised or intuitive systems for making decisions. Unlike Benner, she did not relate this to the experience of the nurses; rather, she saw it as a product of the complexity of the situations they had encountered:

> *The use of decision analysis may not lend itself to analysing and understanding the work of nurse practitioners in general practice. The*

'messiness' of reality in the clinic means that nurse practitioners need to develop the ability to cope with the uniqueness, uncertainty and conflict inherent in real problems. (Offerdy, 1998: 999).

Rationality and decision making

This emphasis on describing and analysing nurses' decisions underpins a number of recent studies. Following Benner, there has been a continued interest in the role of intuition in nurses' decisions (for a review see Cioffi, 1997). However it is also possible to identify concerns about Benner's approach and her positive evaluation of intuitive decision making. The highly individualistic and virtually invisible aspects of intuitive decision making rest uneasily with moves towards greater professional accountability and therefore a higher level of transparency (see, for example, moves towards clinical governance in the NHS (NHS Executive, 1999: 2–3)). If nurses and other professionals are to account for their decisions then they must be able to show how and why they made a particular decision, demonstrating both the appropriateness of the decision-making process and of the information.

Much attention has focussed on the nature of the information used and there has been considerable pressure to ground decisions within appropriate information. In the health service this has taken the form of evidence-based practice. Luker and Kenrick undertook an exploratory study of the type of information used by 47 community nurses in making their clinical decisions. They identified three types of knowledge which influenced decisions.

The categories generated by the sources of influence data seemed to reflect a descriptive framework which suggested that nurses' clinical decisions were informed by:

1. *knowledge based on research and tested theories,*
2. *knowledge based on practice and arising out of nursing experiences,*
3. *knowledge which is commonsense and current in everyday life.* (Luker and Kenrick, 1992: 459).

Luker and Kenrick's study contained an explicit criticism of Benner's approach. For example, they noted that:

It is little wonder that many community nursing curricula are based on Benner's framework as it seems to account for the experience so valued by practitioners. Whilst we would not devalue clinical experience in any way, we suggest that Benner has popularized the notion of experience at the expense of science. (Luker and Kenrick, 1992: 463).

In many ways this seems to miss the point. Benner was not directly concerned with the substance of specific decisions and therefore with the relevance of specific types of knowledge. She was actually concerned with the process of decision making. In contrast, Luker and Kenrick were interested in the type of information used rather than the decision-making process. They were concerned with identifying and classifying the different types of knowledge which nurses invoke to justify their decisions. Their relative neglect of decision making reflects a narrow rationalistic approach to decision making in which a decision was a product of the identification of appropriate knowledge. This may be a reasonable approach to the process of decision making when issues are simple and relatively straightforward – for example, where the problem is easy to define in an uncontested way, the choices are limited, the benefits or costs of particular courses of action are established and the consequences are limited. However, some decisions are more complex – for example, there may be a wide range of choices, the benefits and costs may not be clear and there may be major consequences for individuals involved. These type of decisions often involved dilemmas.

Values in decision making

Sletteboe has undertaken a conceptual analysis of dilemmas in nursing. Dilemmas were associated with complex decisions as they involve choices between negative consequences: in some cases the potential negative outcomes were so serious that the dilemma was associated with high-risk or fateful decisions, which Sletteboe referred to as 'life and death' decisions (Sletteboe, 1997: 449). Dealing with a dilemma is a distinctive type of decision making, as is clear in Sletteboe's discussion of the attributes of dilemmas (Box 4.1).

Box 4.1 Attributes of dilemmas (Sletteboe, 1997: 449)

- *Equally unattractive alternatives.* There have to be two or more alternatives to choose between, all of which are considered undesirable.

- *Awareness of alternatives.* The moral agent has to know about the alternatives to see the situation as a dilemma. If he or she lacks the knowledge that different alternatives could be chosen, the dilemma is not recognised.

- *Need for a choice.* One has to make a decision and make a choice of one of the alternatives.

- *Uncertainty of action.* The choice to be made is difficult because one does not know the real consequences of the choice or because the consequences are unwanted but unavoidable. One does not know the right thing to do.

Erlen and Sereika (1997) identified the issue of ethical decision making in critical care nursing, which by definition frequently involved high-risk or fateful decisions. They defined ethical decisions as those which concerned nurses' responses to inappropriate treatment:

Nurses in ICUs are often confronted with life sustaining treatment decisions. These decisions centre on the inappropriate use of antibiotics, artificial nutrition, cardio-pulmonary resuscitation and mechanical ventilation, as well as the burdensome nature of these treatment to patients. (Erlen and Sereika, 1997: 953; see also Husted and Husted, 1995).

As Erlen and Sereika pointed out, this type of decision may provoke anxiety and stress for nurses. Underlying the technical aspects of the decisions are issues of values which nurses may not have been trained to deal with:

Stress occurs when nurses try to reconcile their ideals of patient care with what the reality of nursing is. (Erlen and Sereika, 1997: 954).

Given the complexity of the situations nurses deal with and the decisions they make, there has been considerable interest in enhancing nurses' ability to make decisions. Schön (1991) argued that this capacity can be developed through the process of reflecting in and on practice. Reflection involves thinking about situations and decisions both at the time and afterwards so that a nurse can both make better decisions and also learn from the experience of decision making. Since reflective practice is linked to personal and professional development and learning, discussions of reflective practice tend to form part of the general discussion of nurse education. Thus, a major review of reflective practice edited by Palmer and her colleagues did not include either decision making or risk in the index (Palmer *et al.*, 1994). However, in Johns' chapter reflective practice was clearly linked to decision making as forming: for example, the framework which Johns provided to guide the reflective practitioner centered on decision making (Box 4.2).

However, the relevance of reflective practice for nurse decision making has been concealed by a tendency to see reflection as a form of psychotherapy. For example, in the guidance provided by Johns, nurses were invited to reflect on their personal feelings about situations and decisions using the following questions:

How did I feel about this experience when it was happening?
How do I now feel about this experience? (Johns, 1994: 112).

Thus, in accounts of reflective practice, the description and analysis of decisions and risks tends to get lost in and buried by practitioners' analyses of their own feelings and personal reactions (see for example Holm and Stephenson, 1994).

Box 4.2 Decision making in reflective practice (Johns, 1994: 12)

2. Reflection
    2.1 What was I trying to achieve?
    2.2 Why did I intervene as I did?
    2.3 What were the consequences of my actions...
3. Influencing factors
    3.1 What internal factors influenced my decision making?
    3.2 What external factors influenced my decision making?
    3.3 What sources of knowledge did/should have influenced my decision making?
4. Could I have dealt better with the situation?
    4.1 What other choices did I have?
    4.2 What would be the consequences of these choices?

It is important to recognise the psychological tension or anxiety which nurses often experience when they make decisions. Indeed the more complex, fateful and risky a decision the more likely it is to provoke anxiety. In itself anxiety may not be harmful, and mild anxiety may be a positive stimulus to action. Anxiety only becomes harmful when it is so severe that it prevents decisions and actions (Borrill and Bird, 1999) or when the response to anxiety is dysfunctional. For example, Menzies (1970) has argued that many of the negative features of traditional nursing, such as the depersonalisation of the nurse–patient relationship through task-oriented nursing and through the regular movement of nurses between wards, are a dysfunctional defence against anxiety. It is possible to see Benner's analysis of decision making in the same way. 'Novice' nurses are likely to experience higher levels of anxiety and therefore use formalised rule-based decision-making systems as a defence against this anxiety. As nurses acquire experience and confidence they no longer feel the need for the protection offered by such systems and develop more intuitive approaches.

Professionals have to make or to participate in making decisions in conditions of uncertainty, and some of these decisions will have high consequences for their clients. The growing concern with the ways in which professionals make decisions has stimulated a literature on decision making. Benner's analysis of the ways in which nurses develop expertise and confidence in decision making has been influential, although it raised a number of issues. In an environment where the actions and decisions of nurses and other professionals are increasingly subject to scrutiny, it is important that both the process and type of information being used can be externally evaluated. If inexperienced nurses use formalised decision-making systems as a defence against anxiety is it possible to provide them with a more explicit understanding of decision making so that they can use more functional approaches? It is clear that the type of insight which they require can only come from an analysis of the sorts of decisions involving nurses and it is to this we turn in the remainder of this chapter.

STUDYING NURSING DECISION MAKING

Although there is interest in the ways in which nurses make decisions, most of the existing research is not particularly helpful. It either compares actual decision making with some ideal, as in Luker and Kenrick's study (1992); invites nurses to comment on *hypothetical* decisions, as in both Sletteboe's (1997) and Erlen and Sereika's (1997) studies; or the prime focus is on the ways in which nurses develop their expertise to make decisions rather than on the decisions themselves, as in Benner's study (1984). We want to supplement this literature by exploring the actual nature of decisions.

To examine the nature of decision making we needed to capture 'real' clinical decisions and then to explore the characteristics of different types of decisions. One way of 'capturing' decisions is to actually observe them and we did undertake observation of decision making in multidisciplinary teams (which we discuss in Chapter 5). However, observation is both labour intensive and intrusive. We decided to use a less intrusive approach to capturing decision making. We asked participants to act as observers and to record their observations in diaries. We were following the approach of Zimmerman and Wieder (1977) in which they used diaries plus follow-up interviews:

> *Individuals are commissioned by the investigator to maintain ... a record over some specified period of time according to a set of instructions .... The technique we described emphasizes the role of diaries as an observational log maintained by subjects which can then be used as a basis for intensive interviewing.* (Zimmerman and Wieder, 1977: 481).

The approach contained three elements: an initial interview, the research diary and a debriefing interview. The initial briefing interview was not only used to explain to diarists how we wanted them to complete their diaries; we also used it to explore the participants' views of risk and risk learning. At the end of the formal interview each participant was given a diary. This was designed to capture some of the decisions and situations in which the participant was involved, in clinical practice, so that the risk and learning implications could be explored in a debriefing interview. Thus, diarists were invited to record for each shift the general activities that took place plus two decisions which they made during the shift. The diarists were not given a structured format but were invited to make their own record for each shift. As guidance, they were provided with a set of written instructions and at the end of the initial interview, the researcher explained how to fill them in and arranged to visit the diarist after completion of one entry so that she could review the entry and supply additional guidance if necessary.

Following our experiences in an ESRC project (Alaszewski *et al.*, 1998), we decided to concentrate on decisions rather than risk. In that project, diarists had been invited to complete a diary to record incidents which had risk implications. They tended to record critical incidents, i.e. high consequence incidents, and more mundane decisions tended to be omitted. Benner (1984) also found that:

> *With experience we learned that the research term, 'critical incident,' was an unfortunate label because it triggered thoughts of critical patients and crisis events. We had to explain that we were interested in significant non crisis events as well.* (Benner, 1984: 16).

The number of entries depended on the particular work pattern and, for students, the nature and length of their placement. Generally, the research team aimed to have at least 10 complete entries, though in one or two cases it was only possible to obtain five entries: however, this still ensured that each diarist identified at least 10 decisions, and some substantially more.

When the participant had completed the agreed number of entries, the researcher collected the diary. The researcher undertook a preliminary analysis of the diary and identified and classified decisions. Once this had been completed the researcher selected two contrasting decisions. These then formed the basis of the debriefing interview. The researcher explored with respondents how and why the decision had been made, their involvement in the decision, the risk implications of the decision, the extent to which they had been prepared for the decision and the teaching and learning implications of the decision.

In ethnographic research, cases are not selected in terms of their representativeness of some defined population but rather in terms of their relevance for the purpose of the research. Since we were interested in community nursing for three different client groups, we decided to include in our study nurses whose practice was predominately oriented to each client group: learning disability nurses, community mental health nurses and nurses working with older people.

We adapted Benner's typology of practitioners to select practitioners with different levels of competence within each professional group. Although Benner was primarily concerned with hospital nursing, whereas we are interested in nursing in the community, her work was appropriate for our study. Not only did she use a similar ethnographic approach to data collection, interviews plus observation but her typology was based primarily on competence in decision making. For example, she used a risk-related category, critical incidents, as one of the main instruments of her study and suggested that the main defining characteristic of expert practitioners was their intuitive grasp of clinical situations which related to their skill in decision making:

> Intuitive grasp   *Direct apprehension of a situation based upon a background of similar and dissimilar situations and embodied intelligence or skill ...*   Intuitive grasp *makes expert human decision making possible.* (Benner, 1984: 295).

Benner defined five levels of competence: novice, advanced beginner, competent, proficient and expert. Although Benner's study was concerned to identify the particular characteristics of each type of practitioner, she initially defined novices as newly graduated nurses and experts as nurses with 5 years of clinical experience. In our study we were concerned with the impact of training, so our first group were *advanced students*, i.e. students in the last year of their training. Our second group were *inexperienced practitioners*, which was similar to Benner's novice group. It was made up of newly registered nurses who had been qualified for less than 1 year. Our third and final group, *experienced practitioners*, covered Benner's proficient and expert categories as they possessed at least 3 years of clinical experience. We included 20 diarists in the study. Since there is no specialist registration for care of older people, we included both nurses undertaking the adult branch training and district nurse training, although given the difference in background between district nurse students and other students, we analysed data from their diaries separately. We included two diarists in each category. Thus the sample included 20 diarists: 8 students, 6 newly qualified practitioners and 6 experienced practitioners.

The use of diaries plus debriefing enabled us to capture decisions and to examine a sample of those decisions in more detail. Although the research team provided guidance for the diarist on the nature of decisions, the actual selection was left to individual diarists.

THE NATURE OF DECISION MAKING

In this section we consider the overall pattern of decision making and in the next section we examine in more detail a series of decisions which were identified in diaries and subsequently formed the basis of debriefing interviews.

Identifying and classifying decisions

We asked all diarists to identify at least two decisions which they made during each shift. Despite this request some diarists did not differentiate between decisions and the other activities which they recorded. Therefore we analysed the text of each diary to identify the decisions made by the diarist. We used choice as our criterion for identifying decisions. If the nurse had a choice, then either implicitly or explicitly he or she had made a decision. This can be seen in the following extract that describes a therapy session which the user rejected. The mental health nurse had the choice to terminate the therapy sessions but decided not to:

Assessment of Mr Smith who is known to me over the years. He has drug/alcohol problems, is impulsive and borderline learning difficulty. He wants help with stress but becomes angry and walks out of the session. This is not unusual, I do not respond but leave his case open till next time.

For the purpose of this book, we re-examined all the diaries and identified 584 decisions in the 20 diaries completed by nurses. (In our initial analysis we had identified 528 decisions; the extra 56 decisions came from a careful re-examination of all the activities identified in the diaries.)

We then examined each of these decisions in terms of its apparent focus or purpose, who participated in making the decision and how the decision was made. We will discuss each aspect of decision making in turn.

Focus of decision making

Given the subject matter of the diaries and the main activities of the diarist, it was hardly surprising that the prime focus or purpose of decisions was the provision of care and support (Table 4.1). The overwhelming majority of decisions were concerned with care for individual service users (464, 80%). The following extract from an experienced mental health nurse's diary describes a client-focussed decision:

Risk assessment on short stay ward for a middle aged lady who had taken an overdose due to relationship problems – decided that she did not present a risk of further self harm, and that she did not need to engage with the mental health services.

The second most important single category could be linked to the decision maker's personal development or welfare (49 decisions, 8%). Some diarists decided to undertake an activity or course of action because it provided them with an opportunity for learning. This type of decision making was particularly prominent among student nurses (28 decisions, 21%). For example,

Table 4.1 The focus of decision making (value in per cent)

	Client care	Carer support	Other providers	Self	Agency	Public	Multiple
Older people							
n = 274	80	—	1	9	1	—	9
Mental Illness							
n = 160	83	1	2	9	1	—	4
Learning disability	75	1	4	5	1	1	13
n = 113							
Students							
n = 131	69	—	4.5	21	1	—	4.5
District nursing students							
n = 62	89	—	—	3	2	—	6
Inexperienced							
n = 198	86	2	2	4	—	—	6
Experienced							
n = 193	77	—	—	7	—	—	15
Allt							
n = 584	80	1	2	8	1	—	9

one student working on a ward for the care of older people asked if she could feed a patient so that she could gain experience with this clinical procedure:

One decision I made during this shift in relation to patients was to ask the nurse if I could feed 'Dorothy' [pseudonym] via her gastronomy tube. I have done this procedure once before but it was about 1 year 3 months earlier.

Among the decisions made by experienced nurses we also identified some which concerned the nurses' own situation, but these tended to be related to the nurses' work load or safety. Thus, one experienced district nurse noted her decision to raise the nature of the work load and activities in response to the team leader's statement that the work load of the team was to increase:

Meeting at 12 with our Team manager. We are told that the over 75's service is to be within our remit. [I] advised the manager we have trouble getting reassessments done. Apparently she wasn't aware! It is clear that she doesn't fully understand our role as District Nurses and seems to relate to hospital nurses. [I] had to put forward what we see our role as, and that we just do not go into homes and fill in forms without looking at the patient as a whole. This is taking our accountability to the full, rather than creating face to face contact [to fulfil the conditions of the] GP contract.

This nurse also recorded her concerns about dealing with the verbal abuse from clients whose appointments had to be cancelled because of lack of time and resources.

We found it difficult to identify decisions in the diaries where the prime concern or purpose was the welfare of informal carers or the public or the activities of other service providers or the agency which employed the diarist. This did not mean that the diarists were unaware of the interests or activities of other parties; rather, that they gave precedence to and tended to justify decisions in terms of the service user's interests. This can be seen in the following extract from the diary of an experienced district nurse who decides that she needs to 'facilitate' a decision by the user's GP to visit a patient she was concerned about:

> *Discussion with the GP re one of his patients who, I am very concerned about. After talking the GP also stated 'he had been concerned about this lady', but hasn't visited for a long time. Practically had to 'allow' the GP to make the decision that this lady needs assessment for her mobility. Knowing the GP is an art and how to make them see what is their decision.*

An analysis of the 50 multiple-focus decisions showed that while the the decision maker was primarily concerned with the interests of the service users (49 of the 50 decisions), they were also concerned with the interests of the carers (27 of the 50 decisions). There was also some evidence that nurses considered their own welfare and interests (17 of the 50 decisions) and those of other service providers (7 of the 50 decisions) alongside users' interests. Again, there was little evidence of wider concerns, such as those of the agency (one decision) or the general public (two decisions).

Thus, the interests of carers were considered alongside those of main service users. In the following extract a district nurse student with a case load of older people considered that her client would benefit if his wife undertook the care of his catheter but given her trepidation decided to enhance her skills and confidence slowly:

> *Next chap a regular. Contriving to support wife regarding catheter care although I end up doing all the work; the wife prefers to just watch. I am allowing the wife to accept her responsibilities slowly. If I force her to do something she's not confident or comfortable with we may lose her support altogether.*

Participation

While the interests of service users were the main focus of decision making, there was little evidence of nurses treating users or carers as major partners in the decision-making process (Table 4.2). Nurses appeared to make the

Table 4.2 Participation in decision making (values in per cent)

	Alone	Other provider	User and/or carer	Multiple
Older people n = 274	77	4	1	18
Mental illness n = 160	50	2	1	47
Learning disability n = 113	60	2	1	37
Students n = 131	61	12	3	24
District nursing students n = 62	84	—	—	16
Inexperienced n = 198	66	—	—	34
Experienced n = 193	61	1	—	38
All n = 584	65	3	1	31

majority of decisions by themselves (382 decisions, 65%). This was particularly evident in nurses caring for older people, especially district nurse students. A newly qualified district nurse recorded a decision which could have been made involving the client but she choose to make it on her own:

> Mrs S has on previous visits stated that she is petrified of the procedure resulting from a bad experience, when her blood was taken in hospital. Prior to the visit, I had updated my knowledge on the techniques of venepuncture. Consequently I saw my role in diminishing the risk of fear, as gaining the patient's confidence by my own unhurried, confident manner, explaining the procedure in a way in which she found acceptable and also altering the order in which I carried out the procedure.

It was also possible to identify similar missed opportunities in other diaries. For example, a newly qualified nurse responded to a crisis by making a decision to abandon a treatment plan:

> Client D rang to cancel Day 5 of de-sensitisation plan. Went to home to visit. Very distressed. Decide to abandon plan. Reassess D's needs. Appointment given at the clinic next week.

When nurses did involve other individuals in the decision-making process, it tended to be other service providers, whose expertise they required. This was particularly evident among student nurses, who often referred to their practice teacher or mentor. A student mental health nurse used his practice teacher in the following way:

> *I discussed with R about my doing the assessment re this client. I explained my reticence about conducting it myself and we decided for me to just sit in on this one; this was not discussed with the client – not appropriate/relevant.*

Qualified nurses often needed to involve other professionals in the decision-making process because they had the formal authority or specialist knowledge. A newly qualified mental health nurse recorded her use of a clinical psychologist:

> *Meeting with Eva the Psychologist. I have asked for her advice re client D and client R. This is very useful. Decide to continue with D alone but with new care plan as devised by Eva. Decide to ask R if she will see Eva and I together to look at her phobia in more detail.*

Similarly, an experienced community learning disabilities nurse made use of the client's and general practitioner's expertise:

> *This client lives with adult carers and another two ladies. She attends college and also has respite care. She is at present sexually inactive but is very aware of males and prefers their company. I was previously asked by her Social Worker to liaise with this lady and her GP regarding contraception. Myself and this lady visited the GP and discussed this issue. She refused to have the contraceptive injection and it was felt that oral contraception wouldn't really be feasible due to her learning disabilities etc.*

In some circumstances, nurses did involve a wider group of people in the decision-making process. This was particularly evident in mental health and to a lesser extent in learning disability and also with the more experienced nurses. In some circumstances this was a response to uncertainties and potential harmful consequences of getting it wrong and reflected the 'fateful' decisions that mental health nurses and experienced nurses working in the community have to make. Mental health nurses widened participation to pool information and share responsibility when faced with situations involving low probability/high consequences risks such as suicide. For example, an experienced mental health nurse sought to confirm his judgement that a client was no longer dangerous by calling a multidisciplinary meeting:

> *First appointment with a young man recently discharged from admission ward. I was originally involved in the admission which required Mental Health Act Section 2 services for admission (at that time!) – were 'risk' to others. He attacked his father with a knife. Later he was taken off his*

> *section 'no evidence of mental illness'. My appointment today too confirmed this opinion. Client was asking for discharge. Whilst acknowledging the client's reaction I felt unable to make this decision unilaterally. Accordingly decision made to hold Care Programme Review Meeting.*

However, wider participation also reflected a commitment to 'good practice' and in particular involving users and carers in the decision-making process. This was notably evident within learning disability services and this type of interaction is recorded in the diary of an experienced learning disability nurse:

> *Contacted Ben's parents to ask how things were – stated he was happy at home and appeared OK since leaving residential home. Parents decided that obviously he was unhappy with the environment. Discussed how things were going with finding other placement – parent stated they would continue to chase this up with Social Services. But felt that if they stated that Ben was happy they might not get this. I said that our aim was to ensure he was happy but felt that he would be happier in a smaller house with more activities and that this was a natural transition.*

The process of decision making

In their diaries nurses portrayed themselves as making decisions by themselves in the interests of their clients or patients. They presented a varied picture of the decision-making process. We were able to identify four competing ways in which nurses made decisions:

◆ intuition, using the nurse's own experience and knowledge;
◆ formal, using a structured approach to collecting and using information;
◆ negotiation, in which the decision was reached by discussion between the nurse and another participant; and
◆ meetings, in which the nurse was a participant and shared the decision-making processes with other participants.

The intuitive approach can be seen as the default approach, as the decisions were internalised by the decision maker. There is no external evidence about the nature of the decision making and the decision maker may not be conscious of the decision-making process. This particular approach was particularly evident among learning disability nurses. In the following extract taken from the diary of an experienced learning disability nurse she justified this internal approach by personal knowledge of the client:

> *Decision 2 – To ignore 'testing' behaviour of client 'B'. Client 'B' was knocking on his bedroom wall constantly throughout the night (but intermittently). His mood was calm yet he has a lot on his mind to consider recently. Reassurance offered – 'B' told he could discuss anything he wished*

with staff and that he didn't have to knock on the wall to get our attention. Yet knocking continued so it was ignored as it was safe to do so and he wasn't disturbing anyone else. Decision based on experience of this client; he eventually fell asleep at 5.30 am without incident.

The formal approach required the explicit use of a method for collecting and using information. It was most prominent among nurses providing care for older people, especially district nursing students. It usually involved the use of an explicit method for assessing the service user's condition, such as Orem's model for holistic assessment. This information then formed the basis of subsequent decisions about care and treatment as in the following extract from a district nursing student:

A referral from X Hospital to visit an 89 year old lady who had cancer of the lung. She has been in hospital for 3 weeks with haemoptysis and has a chest drain and radiotherapy. She has a small sloughy wound to her back and a grade 1 pressure sore to her sacrum. Using Orem's model, I assessed this lady but found the only 'nursing' need was that of wound care.

The face-to-face approach was a shared process of decision making and therefore characteristically involved a meeting between the nurse and the other key participants, although in theory the negotiation could have been conducted through some other medium such as a telephone conversation. It was particularly developed among mental health nurses and usually involved the nurse and the service user. The following example is taken from the diary of an experienced mental health nurse but concerns a decision that resulted from face-to-face discussion with the service user's mother:

This gentleman suffers from depression and is on medication to help. He has been seen at the psychiatric clinic which I attend in the past. He has not had a medication review for 2 years and mum feels that he needs one now. I said I would follow it up and contact her with the details.

Meetings also had an element of sharing and often took place when a complex issue or a fateful decision was needed. Experienced nurses were involved in more meetings than other nurses, perhaps because of the greater complexity of the cases that they had to deal with. An experienced mental health nurse noted his use of a team meeting in the following way:

Team Feedback Meeting – I presented two clients to share their potential for aggression/risk to others and agree my strategy.

Benner, in her analysis of decision making (1984), argued that as nurses gain experience and confidence so the pattern of their decision making shifts. Nurses at the start of their career will have little experience and confidence; therefore, Benner argued, they need to use formal structured decision-making processes. As nurses become more experienced and gain more confidence, so the pattern of their decision making changes and increasingly becomes internalised, with increased use of intuition. We could find little evidence to support this analysis in our study. Student nurses predominantly made decisions intuitively and made limited use of formal decision making. Newly qualified nurses made more use of formal approaches but still predominantly used intuition. In the following extract from the diary of a mental health student there is little formal analysis:

> I had been advised to stress to members of the relaxation group that they were there for relaxation and not therapy – any problems to be dealt with by their own key worker. However, after the relaxation techniques have been done, I usually allow 15 minutes at the end to allow members to come out of the deep relaxation before going home. Today the new lady was given some constructive help by the other member who has suffered similar problems in the past and overcome them. It was brought home to me that other sufferers can be very helpful at times and, whereas I could have suggested that talking about problems was not on the agenda, on this occasion I felt the discussion was justified.

Similarly, a newly qualified mental health nurse relied heavily on 'common sense':

> One of my clients is having marital problems and is finding it difficult to cope with an abortion. I definitely feel that we should have more specialisms within the nursing team. No-one has had any training in bereavement counselling which I find astonishing. Luckily my common sense and my client's common sense seem to help us with our sessions which she feels are of benefit.

Experienced nurses made the greatest use of a formal approach and the least of intuition. For example, an experienced mental health nurse based her decision not to provide further sessions for a user who had taken an overdose on a formal risk assessment.

> Risk assessment on 26 year old lady who had taken major overdose at the weekend following long-term 'hassle' from her new husband's former wife. Assessment that she was currently not a high risk of further self harm, but did need further sessions to explore issues, improve stress management.

One explanation for this difference is that Benner's study was conducted in hospital and ours in the community. It is possible that in hospitals as nurses gain seniority they acquire increasing power and there is less need for them to justify their decisions through the use of formal decision techniques. In the community, experienced nurses do acquire seniority but they also appear to take on more complex and riskier cases. Thus, they need the protection provided both by formal approaches and by shared approaches to decision making.

Decision making and associated management of risk is a routine part of everyday nursing practice. Most of the decisions recorded in our nurses' diaries concern client welfare and were made by the nurses themselves. Nurses, especially student nurses, did make some decisions related to their personal development and on occasions were aware of the wider ramifications of their decisions. When making more complex decisions, especially potentially fateful decisions, they tended to involve a wider group. The pattern of decision making varied both between client groups and with the experience of the nurse (Table 4.3). Learning disability nurses presented their decisions as mainly intuitive; nurses caring for older people were more likely to use formal approaches; while mental health nurses placed greater emphasis on face-to-face decision making. We could find little evidence to support Benner's claim that nurses at the start of their careers use predominantly formal methods of decision making and as they become more experienced they increasingly internalise the decision-making process. In our study experienced nurses made least use of an intuitive approach and made the most use of formal decision-making systems and structured meetings. In the next section we examine some nurses' decisions in more depth.

Table 4.3 The process of decision making (values in per cent)

	Intuitive	Formal	Face-to-Face	Meeting
Older people				
n = 274	33	45	19	3
Mental illness				
n = 160	21	31	39	9
Learning disability				
n = 113	42	19	30	9
Students				
n = 131	42	23	30	5
District nursing students				
n = 62	18	56	26	—
Inexperienced				
n = 198	42	28	26	4
Experienced				
n = 193	20	42	26	12
All				
n = 584	32	35	27	6

THE PROCESS OF DECISION MAKING

In the diaries, students and practitioners identified decisions and provided brief descriptions of the nature of the decisions. However, it was often difficult from these accounts to fully understand the decision-making process and to see the decision within context. In the debriefing interviews we were able to explore with diarists two of their decisions. We selected decisions which highlighted specific issues within the diarists' practice so that we could explore the issues in more depth. Since there were 20 nurse diarists, we identified 40 decisions for scrutiny. In this section we select four of these decisions to analyse in more detail. The first decision was one recorded by an experienced learning disability nurse and focusses on an apparently routine decision to provide a user with a training programme. The second decision concerns the dilemma faced by a student nurse when she observed inappropriate behaviour while she was on placement in a nursing home. The third decision was made by an experienced mental health nurse when he decided to monitor a woman who was in a manic stage of her illness. The fourth decision was made by an experienced district nurse and concerns her refusal to recommend an increase in pain relief medication for a terminally ill patient and describes a conflict of interest and of values.

Decision 1   Routine decision made by an experienced learning disability nurse

The first decision selected for more detailed consideration is a relatively routine decision made by an experienced learning disability nurse to provide a young man with severe learning disabilities with a training programme. As with many individual decisions it formed part of a larger complex of decisions which started with the nurse's assessment that the young man's need was for an educational placement. This then led to a process of identifying and choosing a placement. Since the selected placement was in a neighbouring town, it involved a long journey and the nurse decided to provide a training programme to ensure that the young man could reach his new placement safely (Box 4.3).

The training programme formed part of an overall strategy to provide the young man with access to further education. He had previously attended a further education college in the town where he lived but he had stopped going because he did not feel accepted. His learning disability nurse helped him identify an alternative which involved a lengthy journey and therefore decided to support him by providing him with specific training to make the journey:

Box 4.3 Experienced learning disability nurse's decision

Context

Provision of training programme to enable a young man with learning disabilities to access a new educational placement safely.

Decisions

i.   To find a new placement.
ii. Selection of placement.
iii. Provision of training programme.

I chatted with him about what the problems were with [his original placement] and the problem area really was the fact that he felt isolated because of his disability; he was aware of that to an extent and he felt that people ridiculed him. So we talked about actually working and being in a smaller group, whether he would be better suited to that; he wasn't really forthcoming; he said that he preferred that, but he was very cagey, obviously he didn't want [it to fail again] ... he had been at home for several years and spent a lot of time with his mum and subsequently he was very apprehensive of change, so what I did was to actually get to know him really and introduce myself and chat to him, with him coming down here to see me just so that he could get out of the house. I took him out and what we did was visit some places that he could actually go to, and just really got his personal opinion about them ... we got an interview at Market Town College where the lady that interviewed us was very pleasant and basically showed him around and introduced him to all the staff that he would be working with, showed him the groups. They were small groups of 6 or 7 people so we got a picture of it ... he was very actually apprehensive of it all ... I did say to him .... 'Let's give it a try and ... I will attend the college with you and it's the first time for me as well. I don't know anyone the same as you so we're in the boat together but at least there's two of us and we can keep each other company,' so he's quite happy with that.

The nurse saw the young man's interest as the main justification for the decision making. For example, he justified the training programme in the following way:

personally I feel that it's his safety really ... in situations like crossing the road .... I'm aware that he goes in to Kingsport on his own and he does obviously have road sense and does use public transport but you still are never 100% sure so ... the period from leaving the home to returning to home is an assessment period for me. So personally I felt responsible for him; obviously I'm not going to walk off and leave him and say, 'Right I'm going home now, off you go to college.'

Although the nurse sought to involve both the user and his mother in the decision making, it was clear that throughout the whole process, he took the lead and tended to inform other participants after he had made his decisions:

Researcher: How long do you envisage your withdrawal period lasting?

Nurse: Probably a month. I'll give it another month. It's really, well, so that I'm certain that he's happy, that he's settled in...

Researcher: Who is responsible for making the decision?

Nurse: What? When I withdraw?

Researcher: Yes.

Nurse: Me – me and the mum, I suppose, really. I will discuss it with the mum obviously and I'll keep the doctor aware of what we're doing. [I made two initial visits to the family] I made the first visit, and the second day the mum actually phoned up in a distressed state; he was basically driving her around the bend with his obsessive behaviour, so I said I'll come round. So I went round straight away. I chatted with them about the behaviour and discussed possible visits to see a psychiatric consultant, and I explained exactly what their role was, because immediately when you mention – mental health and psychiatry – flashing lights go off. So I explained what their role was and that we could look at the possibilities of medication ... I brought that in because its something that we could do immediately. So I wrote a letter then and made a referral to the GP, asking him to refer him to a psychiatric consultant, and I explained the situation – what my input had been up to then – I was intending to write to the GP about looking at getting him into college, but at the time I didn't know if it was going to be a success, so that it would not really have achieved any point at that moment in time ... now I know he's actually happy about going, so what I'll do now is contact the GP and let him know.

In his discussion of the decision-making process, the nurse did not identify any formal approach to decision making and it was clear that the prime function of his meetings with the user and his mother was to 'explain' his decisions:

Researcher: What was your personal involvement in this decision?

Nurse: I suggested it – I suggested the whole thing. I laid it out how I would go about it. [I] explained to the mum, [I] explained to the chap.

The absence of any formal approach to decision making plus the tokenistic use of face-to-face meetings related to the influence of the nurse's assessment of the situation and the values that underpinned this assessment. The nurse had decided that the mother was overprotecting her son and that he should be encouraged to develop more independence, enabling him to leave home and live independently:

Researcher: I suppose the positive outcomes that might come out of it is ...?

Nurse: Yes, he might go on a full-time course, that's what I'm hoping. Basically he's getting out of the house. What I wanted to do is this integration. It is unhealthy for anyone, unless they're a hermit, to remain in the house 24 hours a day, 365 days a year and not actually see anyone apart from the mother. I want to actually get him mixing with people. Really the idea ... is getting him to actually leave home. It's a natural transition at a certain age and I've chatted with him about it but I'm not pushing it. I obviously don't want to upset him and make him nervous about it. When chatting with the mum, she said that several years ago, with the involvement of learning disability services, he was introduced to a children's home where they were told practically to just leave him and not visit for a while and not to be overly concerned about him. If he was upset not to worry about it. I thought, 'what a wrong way of going about things, that's going to upset him', which it did, so he obviously moved straight back home. But I sort of chatted with mum about what's available and what resources were available. What I would actually look at on moving out would obviously be the house that he was moving to and the people that he was living with ... it would be a gradual introduction ... rather than just dumping somebody in there. You've got to look at the issues of compatibility really and that type of thing.

On the surface this decision might appear relatively straightforward – a routine technical decision made in the interest of the user. If the service user was to get to college safely, it seemed reasonable that the nurse should decide to provide him with a training programme. However, more detailed analysis indicated a more complex picture, especially when the decision was placed within the context of the nurse's overall plans for this young man. The decision was grounded within a strong value base and designed to contribute to an overall goal, independent living. It was not at all clear that this goal and

> **Box 4.4** Student nurse's decision
>
> *Context*
> Student nurse caring for a vulnerable resident in a private nursing home.
> *Decision*
> i. Reports to senior nurses that the resident has vomited and clears up as instructed.
> ii. Helps enrolled nurse put resident to bed.
> iii. Observes enrolled nurse doing a manual evacuation; judges that it is unacceptable practice but is unable to intervene effectively to protect the resident.

the value base on which it was founded were shared by the user or his mother. Although the nurse claimed to consult the user, his mother and other participants, this exercise was rather tokenistic and the nurse effectively made the decisions intuitively and there was little evidence that he systematically collected and used information.

Decision 2   Decision made by a student nurse about inappropriate behaviour

While the value issues were implicit in the first decision, they were explicit and central to the decision which we analyse in Decision 2, which was made by a student nurse on placement in a nursing home for older people. The student nurse observed care which was not acceptable by current standards but felt she did not have the authority to take action (for a summary see Box 4.4).

The student nurse became involved in the resident's care when she observed her vomit in the day room. She suggested to the senior nurses that the resident was unwell and should be put to bed and while the resident was being put to bed the enrolled nurse decided to manually evacuate her bowel. The student nurse clearly felt that this was inappropriate behaviour:

> *I suggested we take the lady back to her room, pop her on her bed because she would want to lie down if she was not feeling too well, a bit under the weather. At this point I didn't realise how ill she was. I mean in two weeks I didn't really learn that much about the patient and her condition .... As we were putting her on the bed we happened to discover that she was ready to go to the toilet and the enrolled nurse said that she would do a PR [per rectum] on her. Now I've come across these before; I've heard of them being done but I didn't expect to see what I saw. She actually*

manually evacuated the lady's bowel. She turned around to me at the time and said 'I don't know whether I should be doing this, I don't know whether it's the done thing these days but sometimes you've got to do it'. I said that I thought it was only used as a very last resort and that maybe she could have an enema first. She said that wouldn't work because it wouldn't stay in. She did it manually and the lady was in a lot of pain; she was laying on her side, on the correct side, and she shouted out. I had never heard her shout: even when she was ill she never spoke, she never said anything, but at this point she did cry out quite a lot .... The enrolled nurse did wear gloves. I sat and tried to comfort the lady as much as I could really.

The student nurse felt that the enrolled nurse was responsible for making the decision to undertake the procedure:

Researcher: Who was responsible for making the decision?
Student nurse: At the time it was my decision to take her to her room, and I would have just left her and maybe kept an eye on her, gone in at regular intervals and made sure she wasn't going to be sick any more, but the decision was the enrolled nurse's to manually do it. I mean not even to just leave her and see how she got on herself; that decision was made by the enrolled nurse.

However, she did recognise that there was a secondary decision; she could choose whether or not to take action by being more forceful at the time. Subsequently, she used the incident to increase her own personal knowledge. She did check in a subsequent placement whether the practice was acceptable and confirmed her initial judgement that it was not. Her inaction had, in her own opinion, condoned the unacceptable behaviour:

Researcher: What was your personal involvement in this decision?
Student nurse: Well, I sort of, I'm not going to say I agreed with it but I went along with it. She said 'I'm going to PR this lady, I have to do it manually' and I sort of went yes, well alright OK; so I think in a way, I didn't condone what she did but I thought I'm the student here, this is an experienced enrolled nurse here, she obviously knows what she is doing. But having spoken to other people, I realise it wasn't the right decision which she made.
Researcher: What was your responsibility?
Student nurse: I think, when I look back, I'm hoping I could have said something more .... I don't know if it's illegal but it is classed as abuse .... I know that since I've been here [in a

Researcher:	hospital placement] I've been asked to PR [per rectum] a patient, and I said, 'Do you mean I have to take it all out', and they said, 'No, you just check and see how things are, you don't take anything out.'
Researcher:	Do you think there's any training you could have which would help you with that?
Interviewer:	I think a lot of students get a bad reputation for being 'know it alls' … so you have this worry that you're going to turn round and say, 'I don't think that should be done' that they'll say, 'She's a right one.' You don't want to get a bad reputation in that sense because, at the end of the day, you've got to have a report done about you and you don't want it to be like, 'She's over confident'…. I wish I had done something about it, but I just didn't feel it was my place as a student.

For this student this was clearly a very unsatisfactory experience, despite the UKCC guidelines for professional practice which clearly state that a nurse should report concerns about inappropriate behaviour:

> *You may also have concerns over inappropriate behaviour by a colleague and feel it necessary to make your concerns known. You will need to report your concerns to the appropriate person or authority.* (UKCC, 1999: 21).

The student had at the time not taken opportunities to discuss the incident with course staff nor did she recognise the need for training in the process of decision making – for example, assertiveness training:

Researcher:	Is there any opportunity for you to go back into college and talk about things, you know if you've had an experience?
Student nurse:	Yes, I think there will be. We had critical incident days where we discussed it but I didn't discuss this particular topic. I had another one; but yes there are opportunities, and we do get to speak with our tutors about it and when you do talk about it you find out that other people are having similar experiences, so it seems to be everywhere.
Researcher:	What about assertiveness training. Do you think that would help?
Interviewer:	I consider myself quite assertive anyway; I mean usually. I think that maybe assertiveness training is to not be ashamed of being a student. I mean why shouldn't a student be clued up on modern day practices?

This decision revolved around a clash of values between a traditional enrolled nurse, who saw nursing very much in terms of physical action, and a student nurse, who was clearly concerned about standards of care and felt that the actions taken by the enrolled nurse constituted inappropriate behaviour. The student nurse felt that through her action she had failed to protect the resident from abuse. She had acquired knowledge from the incident but it was not evident that she would be able to apply this knowledge if a similar incident occurred.

Decision 3   Decision made by an experienced psychiatric nurse to monitor the condition of a hyperactive woman who may have taken an overdose

While risk assessment and management were often implicit in the decisions made by nurses caring for older people and for adults with learning disabilities, they were often explicit within the decisions made by nurses caring for and supporting individuals with mental health problems. The third decision was made by an experienced mental health nurse who had to take responsibility for a woman who was creating difficulties in various locations in a small town, especially in the local maternity unit. The woman was known to have mental health problems and was in a manic state and might have taken an overdose. Having assessed the vulnerability and dangerousness of the woman, the nurse decided that she did not pose a serious threat to herself or to others and therefore decided to monitor the situation (for summary see Box 4.5).

The experienced nurse did not have detailed knowledge of the woman and clearly came under pressure from other health service professionals who felt the woman was a threat to herself and to others.

Box 4.5 Experienced mental health nurse's decision

Context

Woman with a known mental health problem causing problems in various locations in a small market town.

Decision

i. To assess the woman's condition, especially the threat she posed to herself and others.
ii. To monitor the situation and set up contingency facilities.
iii. Not to seek legal powers to detain the woman.

Researcher: Can I ask you about the lady who was in an excitable state?
Nurse: If I can recall correctly this was the lady who we had been asked to monitor over the weekend as part of the new CPN [community psychiatric nursing] service, well known to the team in general but not particularly known to me other than just known as a name; apparently she was a manic depressive, literally sort of buzzing round Market town ... at one stage she ended up on the maternity unit and the nurses had retreated to the office. The security man who was there to protect everyone had retreated behind his desk. One of the nurses during the course of the day, a general nurse, felt she may have taken an overdose .... She was very elated, hypo-manic I suppose the term you're looking at; but she was buzzing, she was on a push bike, her legs were going ten to the dozen. I had pursued her virtually all day Saturday.

The nurse had to make a decision in a situation of uncertainty. He was not sure whether the woman had taken an overdose, nor did he feel he had full knowledge of the normal actions of the woman's medication. However, he did not feel that the woman's condition was sufficiently serious to justify use of the powers provided by the Mental Health Act, 1983; therefore, he decided to monitor the situation:

> *and the decision that I had to look at was her mental state and consider had she taken an overdose; and the decision I made was that I didn't feel she had and I had to let her carry on buzzing around Market town. And I felt my choices were a bit, well I don't think I had many choices, because we felt there was no grounds for mental health sectioning and also I felt that her presentation hadn't changed throughout the day when I had seen her two or three times. But I suppose the thing that strikes you at the end of that decision is 'what if ....' I wonder, and then what, and I think it then makes you question your knowledge of that type of particular medication that she is on; then I started to think about how you've got to update yourself, and nobody tells you to update on what which I think is open to abuse. And I felt that perhaps I needed to update myself more on that particular type of medication.*

The nurse clearly felt that he was responsible for making the decision. Although he recognised the risks posed by the woman, he sought to manage them by balancing her interests with those of the public:

Researcher: Who was responsible for making the decisions?
Nurse: On the day me.
Researcher: And what was your responsibility?

Nurse: I think my responsibility was to the public at large, if that doesn't sound too dramatic, and certainly the lady I don't feel was in a 100% position to advocate for her self for her own risks. I think it was more a case of risk assessment and risk management, two slightly different issues. I was also conscious about creating a management situation out of maybe being, I'm struggling for the right choice of words, but maybe by being too cautious then we would have certainly had a management problem on our hands with the lady without a doubt.

In making his decision the nurse used his experience and intuition:

Researcher: And was there a structured way for making the decision?
Nurse: No, I don't think structured in the sense of having a tool or whatever. I think we had to deal with the situation at the time; it wasn't a nurse/patient relationship in an ideal world where somebody is in bed waiting for you and transferring information; it was managing a situation.
Researcher: Had your training prepared you for making this decision?
Nurse: I think I'd like to say yes, but perhaps the training I received for that sort of decision was maybe some years back; the experience that I have allowed me to make that decision. Being a Community Psychiatric Nurse [you have] a more autonomous decision-making role as opposed to when I was on the wards. When you're an on-call CPN you've got to make some quite potential far-reaching decisions at strange hours and in strange situations so I don't think the situation was totally alien to me.

The nurse recognised that his assessment of the risks was not shared by other health professionals, especially the staff in the maternity unit, but felt that his judgement was based on more specialist knowledge and a desire to avoid creating a sense of panic:

The staff in the maternity unit] were involved purely because this lady had descended on them and I think they were ready to press alarm bells. The call had come through to my department and we acted appropriately. I think they felt supported, because from the time we had received the phone call we were literally with them within 5 or 10 minutes later, so we hadn't left them there. I think they were a bit taken back by our casual approach, our casual attitude to the lady, but I think that was vital. We did go back and talk to the general nurses about the decision we'd made and why. I wouldn't say we gave them education but I think we did give them a bit of

*an education about this lady's condition and how to manage her. I think
they appreciated that .... I felt we had a management situation to handle;
we had relationships we had to try and keep intact. She told me she hadn't
taken an overdose, so I also had to give that some credence and some value.
I also felt my assessment was better than the general nurse's assessment who
was only looking at the behaviour. I saw the behaviour as something not as
alien, like the general nurse did.*

Although his assessment and decision was based on an evaluation of both
information and of benefits of different outcomes, the nurse underplayed
the value element of the process and emphasised the 'objectivity' of his
judgement:

*I suppose personally you do have to make decisions and try to manage
something as best as you see fit. I suppose there were benefits to knowing
her personally, but I suppose my assessment was as objective as I could
make it; maybe that adds value as well.*

The nurse did not feel that he had received much support in reaching the
decision. Although the woman had been seen by other health professionals
involved in her care and the nurse used information provided by them, there
was little evidence that he had involved them in his decision:

Nurse: I think I had made the decision on my own but I knew she
             had been seen by a Social Worker a few days before and a
             Consultant Psychiatrist plus her GP on that day so I knew
             there were no grounds for sectioning; but I made the
             decision regarding what if she had taken an overdose.
Researcher: Were you supported in your decision?
Nurse: Yes, there was another senior sister with me, but I sort of
             got the impression that she'd really left the final decisions to
             me .... I was aware that my colleague had left the decisions
             to me.

Given the different assessments of risk, the nurse making the decision clearly
experienced some anxiety and personal threat:

Researcher: But it affected you didn't it?
Nurse: Yes it affected me in that it made me doubt I suppose: made
             me doubt and question my own decision, outcomes of
             decision, responsibility, accountability, who would back you
             up if ... well, yes, it makes you doubt but maybe that's not
             such a bad thing because I suppose you should question
             your decisions [in] reflected practice .... I think I did feel
             competent, but if you have an arrogant attitude that my

decision is always right I think that's wrong. I think if you don't question your decision I think that's wrong. I think it's just doubts that spring to mind, but sometimes I find I don't get the answers or I get other 'ifs', 'buts' and 'maybes'.

It is clear that this experienced nurse had to make a decision that could have significance with limited and conflicting information. He used his personal experience to assess and balance the risk and decided to monitor the situation. He rejected the pressure to take a more interventionist approach on the basis of his own assessment of the woman's condition and her interests.

Decision 4   Decision made by an experienced district nurse involving a conflict of interests and values

From an early stage in their training, district nurses deal with complex issues. The main change evident in the diaries was a changing level of responsibility. Experienced nurses worked with General Practitioners, and their advice and guidance had considerable influence over the decisions made by GPs. In the following example (Box 4.6) we have selected a case in which the GP had formal and legal responsibility for deciding how much morphine a dying patient should receive, but the district nurse effectively controlled the decision-making process through her control over the provision of information and close working relationship with the GP.

The district nurse described the context of the decision in the following way:

I had a lady who was 95 and was in residential care; she had just deteriorated following a chest infection, which in some respects should have taken her there and then. But she rallied round – it wasn't so much the antibiotics, because she was left a couple of days without them, – but she rallied round; she then deteriorated again about a week after that and she wasn't mobile. She was getting quite frail and she began to develop pressure sores, which were also adding to her problems. Following that, it was

---

Box 4.6 Experienced district nurse's decision

Context

A terminally ill woman with pressure sores and chest infection.

Decision

i.   To place patient on a syringe driver for pain control.

ii. Refusal of request from residential home manager to increase dose of morphine.

decided because the pressure sores were deteriorating ... that she should be put on a syringe driver.

Following this initial decision, the district nurse came under pressure from the manager of the home to increase the amount of morphine being supplied. In her view, this was to participate in an assisted death:

The manager related it [the decision] to the family. [They] were amazed she was still hanging around when she should have died a couple of weeks back. I think the manager [articulated the family's needs] by saying, 'well I'll ask the District Nurse to go put [up the dose in] the syringe driver'. Which makes it sound as though if we up it we'll [be doing] something. Now I had to put my foot [down] by saying 'no sorry the syringe driver is there to make her comfortable and that's what it is doing'. So there was quite a lot of pressure to try and instigate [an increase in dose] but I think we've got to look at the needs of the patient rather than the needs of the people around us. Nothing is ever said directly [about assisted death].

The district nurse conveyed the request to the GP with the information that the current dosage was adequate, in her opinion, for pain relief. The GP based his decision on her advice:

Researcher: Who was responsible then for the decision not to increase the [dose]?

Nurse: The GP – we went back to the GP to discuss it and the GP was working in accordance with us ... because obviously the information he was getting was from us ... well he did go and see the patient and [agreed] 'yes it didn't warrant it' at that time. Come 24 hours later 'yes it did', but obviously at the moment in time – no. I think not so much for myself; but my other colleagues who are D grades got quite a lot of flack about the lady concerned from the manager, not so much [from] the family. She [the manager] was doing a mediator's job between the family, because we never saw them. The other issue ... was the [patient's] daughter was working in the health service.

This nurse felt that the patient's interest was central to her actions and hinted at the underlying ethical issues, but it was clear that these were never openly discussed.

Researcher: What were the anticipated consequences of not increasing it [the dose]?

Nurse: Well there wasn't [any].

Researcher: Were you anticipating any consequences?

Nurse: ... Well the [residential] home side of it ... I don't particularly feel that's my issue. My priority is to the patient. The family can be supported because it was indicated to them, through the manager, that if they could do so ....

Researcher: What were the potential outcomes – positive or negative?

Nurse: From what respect, from the patient?

Researcher: Yes.

Nurse: The positive side that I see is that we did keep the patient pain free because obviously within 24 hours it was reviewed and there was a necessity to up the dose so I feel that we did give the patient ... the problem occurs obviously when we're looking at an age group that people think well as ... you wouldn't do it to a dog and I think we've got ... as practitioners to be seen to be humane in what we are doing. Positive side for me was I felt I was doing the best for the patient; now we're talking about an elderly, frail 95 year old lady.

The nurse in this case felt that the main skills involved in managing this situation were communication skills and that these types of skills could only be acquired through experience in the job:

I don't think in hospital or in training [they prepare you to make this type of decision]. It's having the knowledge of people ... how people react in different situations .... I think you learn that through experience ... if you haven't got the experience behind you you could be waylaid ... you could have looked at that manager being there 24 hours [so you think] she knows best, but I had to draw on my experience ... well there's some training in there to do with pain control .... I think experience allows you to be able to override what the manager was saying .... I think communication skills need to be high [on training agenda]. You can't read out of books how people react in different situations, possibly you can do that with role play, in scenarios ... things like videos ... reading it out of books ... it's not the same as when you're in the situation.

Although this situation involved complex ethical issues and a conflict of interests, it was interesting to note that when asked about the training implications of the decision, the nurse saw these in technical terms, improved communication. Improved communication would only make the ethical issues clearer, it would not resolve them.

COMMENT

Although routine decision making predominates in practitioners' diaries, it is evident that from the earliest stage of their training, nurses are involved in complex and often challenging decisions. It is clear that they place a high priority on their patients' or clients' interests and try to make the 'best decision'. However, most practitioners are self-taught decision makers and believe they can improve the quality of their information by getting better information. Information is important for decision making but there are other components; in particular, all decisions should be grounded in values as they should be designed to achieve a better situation. As Dowie (1999) argued, decisions require both information, about the probability of certain outcomes, and value systems, which need to be used to assess the desirability of different outcomes. He gives a hypothetical analysis of the choices facing nursery rhyme character Humpty Dumpty (Fig. 4.1).

Any decision tree is one possible model of a decision. That drawn up by Humpty's consultant sets out two options as Sit on the Wall (top Branch) and not Sit on the Wall. There are three uncertainties on the top subtree .... Each of the uncertainties must be quantified .... Five outcomes are produced by these scenarios .... Humpty's strengths of preferences for the outcome states had to be quantified in terms of their 'utilities' (desirabilities) for him. (Dowie, 1999: 44).

This analysis does not 'make' the decision; it is merely a way of making the issues clear. In Dowie's example, the consultant's preferred option would have been for Humpty to sit on the wall, but as events turned out it would have

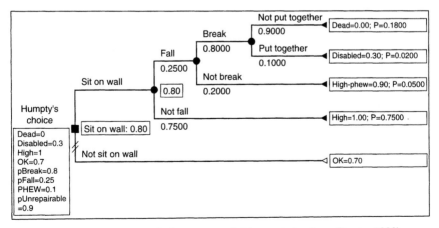

Figure 4.1   Humpty Dumpty's decision tree (with permission from Dowie, 1999).

been better for Humpty if he had not decided to sit on the wall. However, it is clear that decisions are grounded both in available information and the decision maker's value system. Value-free decision making or risk management are contradictions in terms, and therefore nurses should be explicit about the ethical basis of their decision making. We will return to this issue in our concluding chapter.

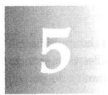

Risk, decisions and teamwork

Helen Alaszewski   Andy Alaszewski

INTRODUCTION

In Chapter 4 we considered risk from the perspective of the individual nurse and his or her decision making. In this chapter we develop our analysis by considering the collective or interprofessional and interdisciplinary aspects. In the first section we examine the ways in which interprofessional working has developed to deal with situations that are complex and where the consequences of incorrect decisions are high, such as child protection or the discharge of mentally ill patients from hospital. In the second section we consider the ways in which nine multidisciplinary teams actually work, exploring in section four the types of decisions which individual practitioners make and the decisions which are made by the team. In the final section we summarise and comment on our analysis.

THE CHANGING PATTERNS OF SERVICES AND PRACTICE

Interdisciplinary work is increasingly considered important and the problems of service coordination exist at practice, agency and policy levels. In this section we examine the development of multiprofessional and multidisciplinary practice as a mechanism for enhancing coordination between services, which ensures that vulnerable clients living in the community do not slip though the health and welfare net.

The coordination problem

Initial identification of the problem

With the establishment of the welfare state in the 1950s, it seemed that the government could provide a comprehensive package of welfare for its citizens, through welfare agencies such as the National Health Service. However, in the 1960s and 1970s, the rising costs of these services, the changing health and welfare needs of the population and the poor quality of some services resulted in a major debate about the nature of welfare provision. Most of the criticism focused on the nature of administrative structures of welfare agencies. These were small and fragmented and, as a result, service users did not receive an integrated package of services. There appeared to be little cooperation between the various professional groups involved in the delivery of services.

This concern with coordination was one of the major stimuli to the restructuring of welfare services in the 1970s which included the formation of local authority social services departments in 1971 and the formation of an integrated NHS in 1974. These different services were expected to cooperate with each other. For example, local authority personal social services departments, which were designed to provide social care for vulnerable individuals in an area, shared the same boundaries as health authorities which provided health care.

These restructurings did not solve the coordination problem; indeed, they may have reinforced it. Local agencies tended to be grouped around the skills of key service providers – for example, social services around social workers and the health service around doctors and nurses. Thus, the needs of individual vulnerable users continued to be provided by a range of specialist agencies.

There is general commitment to coordinating the activities of welfare agencies. As Wildavsky has pointed out, coordination has become so widely accepted that it is 'one of the golden words of our time' and service providers generally accept the principle that they 'should contribute to a common purpose at the appropriate time and in the right amount to achieve co-ordination' (Wildavsky 1979: 132). Wistow and Fuller (1983), in a national survey of collaboration, found that authorities were committed to the principle of integrated services and to teamwork at practitioner level (see also Booth, 1981;

Glennerster *et al.*, 1983a, 1983b). In reality, coordination seems difficult, if not impossible, to achieve.

If organisations shared the same objectives and operated through similar processes, then coordination should be relatively easy. But where organisations differ in their objectives and have different structures and processes then, as Harrison and Tether (1987) have pointed out, coordination is not collaboration but coercion. One organisation must dominate and change the other.

More recently, Hudson (1999a, 1999b) has outlined four major barriers to collaborative teamwork which continue to inhibit joint working across the health/social care divide. These include:

◆ different patterns of employment and accountability in health and social services;
◆ different approaches to and structures for making decsions;
◆ different models for distributing resources;
◆ different professional cultures.

Failure to coordinate

In many areas of health and social care, there has been evidence that professionals and agencies failed to coordinate their actions and that clients were suffering as a result. For example, Skeet (1970) identified the consequences for older people of the failure to effectively coordinate hospital and community services and these problems persist. Means and Smith summarised the situation in the following way:

> *Recent research has pointed to major inadequacies in discharge arrangements for those [older people] returning to their own homes. It was found, that of 60 elderly people discharged from hospital back to their homes, 'One in three of the people in the sample said they had not been asked how they would manage at home after their discharge. Two fifths were told about the discharge either the day before or on the day it was due to happen'.* (Means and Smith, 1994: 156).

Some of the earliest and most persistent difficulties have been evident in the field of child protection and we will consider these as they have had a key influence on the whole debate.

Since the publication of the report of the committee of inquiry into the death of Maria Colwell (Secretary of State for Social Services, 1974), there has been a stream of child abuse inquiry reports. Most inquiry teams were directed to examine the coordination of services and most identified the failure to coordinate the activities of different agencies and professionals as a major factor in the failure to protect some children from abuse. A Department of

Health and Social Security (DHSS) team reviewing these reports described the coordination problems in the following way:

> *The reports demonstrate that problems can arise where there is lack of clarity about the different contributions of the various agencies and individuals involved. Problems can also arise when a particular worker is asked to fulfill several different roles which are not clearly distinguished. Finally there are problems of overlap where particular functions are held in common by more than one agency.* (DHSS, 1982: 5).

Although the legal responsibility for protecting children rests with social services, a whole range of agencies and professionals may have contact with a particular child and may have information relevant to the care and protection of the child. In the 18 reports examined by the DHSS, 24 different kinds of professional and voluntary workers were mentioned. Problems arose when these professionals did not share their information and agree or accept joint decisions. In its review the DHSS noted that there was a tendency:

> *when many people have duties in relation to one family, for responsibility to become blurred and decisions avoided and for vital information to be lost sight of or overlooked.* (DHSS, 1982: 17).

These problems persisted into the 1980s. For example, the inquiry chaired by Lord Justice Butler-Sloss (1988) was appointed as a result of public concern about 'an unprecedented rise in the diagnosis of child sexual abuse during the months of May and June 1987 in the County of Cleveland' (Butler-Sloss Inquiry, 1988: 1). The inquiry was particularly concerned with a 'fundamental breakdown in communication with and co-operation between various disciplines which was impeding the proper approach to the care and protection of children' (Butler-Sloss Inquiry, 1988: 1).

In the 1990s similar problems have been identified in the care and support of individuals who have an enduring mental illness. Within mental health policy the inquiry into the killing of Jonathan Zito by Christopher Clunis also highlighted the failure of professionals and agencies to share information and coordinate activities (Ritchie Report, 1994). Under Section 117 of the 1993 Mental Health Act, health authorities and social services authorities have a duty to provide aftercare for patients who had been detained under Section 3 of the Act. Failures of coordination meant that Christopher Clunis slipped through the gaps between agencies with disastrous consequences. This inquiry is particularly relevant for this research because it identified risk as a central issue. The failure to pool information resulted in a failure to identify the threat which Christopher Clunis presented. The inquiry's report stimulated the Department of Health to review arrangements for interagency working for the care and protection of mentally ill people:

A consistent theme of reports published in the last two years, both on mental health in general and on individual cases, has been the need for greater co-ordination on the part of different agencies which play a part in caring for severely mentally ill people in the community. This is a concern shared by the Department of Health, and following the publication in 1994 of the Report into the Care of Christopher Clunis *work was set in hand to produce detailed guidance on the subject.* (Department of Health, 1995: para 1.1).

Responding to the problem

Rationality versus incrementalism

There has been considerable debate among academics and policy makers about the best way of overcoming the problem of coordination. The debate about coordination is very similar to the debate about decision making which we explored in Chapter 4. It is possible to identify two approaches: in one, the emphasis is on improving decisions through the use of more rational techniques; and the other involves a more pragmatic approach.

Advocates of the rational approach see policy making as a 'top-down' process, with policy makers at the top defining the aims and objectives of service provision and by implication dealing with issues of values. Front-line staff then 'implement' policies, making technical or rational decisions designed to achieve overall organisational aims and objectives. Faludi, in his discussion of planning, established an explicit link between rational decision making and coordination between agencies. He argued for the introduction of multi-planning agencies, or:

agencies with an overlapping action space attempting to continuously coordinate what they are doing with a cumulative rationalising effects so that one may see 'comprehensive planning' as a process. (Faludi, 1973: 208)

In the rational approach, the problem of coordination is seen as essentially a technical problem, usually a lack of appropriate information resulting from inadequate systems of communication. The failure of individual professionals to coordinate their actions is seen as a failure of communication. Agencies need to create structures to ensure effective communication both within and between agencies.

This rational model of organisation coordination found favour in the 1970s and can clearly be seen in the emphasis on structures and planning as mechanisms of coordination. For example, the working party on collaboration between the health service and social services saw joint planning as a method of improving the communication between the two services:

The real objective (of joint planning) is not to achieve joint considerations
of plans prepared separately ... rather [it is] to secure genuinely
collaborative methods of working throughout the process of planning, and
close and continuing co-operation between the officers of the two sides.
(DHSS, 1973).

The rationalist approach has its critics. Lindblom argued that its emphasis on information can be self-defeating; the cost of obtaining comprehensive information may outweigh the anticipated benefits. He compares it to pulling up a tree to gain information about its roots. Furthermore, some problems cannot be resolved by rationality. For example, more information will not resolve a conflict over aims and objectives which is the product of different value systems. Some 'communication' failures are in fact a product of precisely such value conflict: for example, in the 1970s, failures in child protection cases were often associated with different emphases on the rights of parents to autonomy and rights of children to protection (Corby, 1996: 14).

Lindblom (1979) suggested an alternative approach to both decision making and service coordination – incrementalism. Incrementalism is essentially pragmatic: it avoids fundamental reviews of all options, the rationalistic approach, but it also avoids fundamental reviews of aims and underpinning values; instead, it concentrates on the practicalities of decision making and particularly on the available room or 'increment' for change. Both the overall direction of development of policy and the nature of information required are identified as part of the decision-making process. This can be clearly seen in interactions between organisations in decision making, which Lindblom termed partisan mutual adjustment.

Lindblom (1965) argued that agencies operating in the same locality often had different aims and competed over resources. However, for individual agencies there were advantages in collaboration if they could find common ground with other agencies. Through adjustments in areas that were not critical to the agency, it could ensure that its critical aims were achieved. Thus, agencies could adjust their activities through a process of bargaining and negotiation:

Agencies are 'partisan' in that they pursue their own interests but they are
capable of 'mutual adjustment', in that they adapt to the decisions made by
other agencies, or attempt to influence them through negotiation,
bargaining and manipulation. (Harrison and Tether, 1987: 82).

The policy response to the coordination problem has been very much within the technical/rationalist tradition, with the prescription of structures based on the top-down coordination of services. Given the prominence of child protection, this approach has been developed within this area. In 1986, the DHSS issued draft guidance (DHSS, 1986) which prescribed a two-tier coordinating structure and reinforced the lead role of social services in service coordination. The Joint Child Abuse Committee (JCAC) was the top tier. The committee was to include officers from all the major agencies involved in child abuse and was an interagency forum for 'developing, monitoring and reviewing child abuse policies and how they are working' (DHSS, 1986: 28).

At practice or front-line level, the DHSS endorsed the use of case conferences as an 'essential feature of interagency co-operation' and as a forum 'for the exchange of information between professionals involved with the child and family'. The DHSS felt that these conferences allowed for interagency, multidisciplinary discussions and decision making. They recommended that case conferences should be supplemented by other mechanisms of coordination, especially by a key worker. The key worker, who would be a social worker from either the local authority or the National Society for the Prevention of Cruelty to Children (NSPCC) designated at the case conference, would take on responsibility for 'the professional management of the case'. The key worker would also be 'responsible for maintaining regular contact with other agencies and coordinating the interagency work' and for establishing and maintaining a networking role in the following way:

> *Effective interagency working requires the designation of a key worker to co-ordinate the various agencies' contributions to the assessment, ensure that an interagency plan of action is developed and implemented and that it is regularly reviewed on a multi-disciplinary basis, and to act as a focal point for the communication between agencies.* (DHSS, 1986: 18).

In mental health services the Care Programme Approach (CPA) is based on similar principles. It was developed in response to the coordination and communication problems identified in 'community care tragedies' (Reith, 1998). The CPA keyworker has overall responsibility for coordination, monitoring and review.

Researching coordination

In the 1970s and 1980s researchers became dissatisfied with the somewhat artificial distinction between rationality and incrementalism (Smith and May, 1993). In particular there was concern about the polarisation between the central managerial control, implicit in rational models, and the *laissez-faire* policy drift and local autonomy of the incremental model. Researchers' interest has developed in examining the actual process of inter-organisational interaction and several major research findings have emerged: the differences in participants' objectives and value systems; the importance of networks; and the role of resources.

In both the rational and incremental models, organisations form the main unit of analysis and are treated as if they had objectives and value systems. Smith and Cantley have argued that organisations do not have objectives. Only participants within the organisation – for example, managers, service providers and clients – have objectives and these objectives will vary according to their interests and values (Smith and Cantley, 1985). The objectives of the different participants are related to their different perceptions, or in Young's (1977) term 'assumptive worlds', and the various participants have varying abilities or power to impose their definition and to achieve their particular objectives.

Glennerster and colleagues (1983a, 1983b) used this approach to examine collaboration through joint planning between health and personal social services. They interviewed officers in the health service and local government and found that they operated within very different assumptive worlds. NHS officers tended to view planning as a technical exercise and relied heavily on national guidelines and national information. Local government officers tended to see planning as competition between different departments for limited and shrinking resources. They generally disregarded national guidelines and used information as a way of supporting their particular case.

Glennerster and his colleagues showed that it was impossible to understand the nature of collaboration without examining the objectives and intentions of the individuals who were expected to collaborate.

A second major research theme concerns the specific patterns of relations of networks between participants in different organisations. The division between decision making within an organisation and coordination between organisations may be artificial. For some participants their relationship with individuals in other organisations is as important, if not more important, than their relationships in their own organisation. Friend *et al.* (1974) referred to these individuals as reticulists who can use their social networks to coordinate the activities of different organisations.

McKeganey and Hunter (1986) used this approach to examine the coordination of services for older people in one area of Scotland. In this area a team composed of four doctors tried to coordinate the activities of the NHS and local authority services by negotiating patient exchanges between the two authorities.

McKeganey and Hunter argued that the team had a reticulist or networking role: that is, it acted as an arbiter between the different services and enhanced mutual understanding and mutual work. For this role the team members had to appear to be neutral and their success in performing it depended on the *lack* of an organisational base: they were not perceived as being tied to a specific agency. McKeganey and Hunter drew attention to another major variable in inter-organisational relationships: the role of resources and the power relations involved. They argued that the team also had a power-dependency relationship with the social work department. The team could, and did, act on behalf of the social work department.

Hallett's (1995) influential study of interagency coordination found strong support for interagency and collaborative working:

> *Almost unanimously, those interviewed accepted the importance of working together and appeared to value it.* (Hallett, 1995: 295).

She identified three key elements in effective collaboration: clarity over roles, exchange of information and shared decision making. Interagency collaboration is sometimes equated with joint working and Hallett noted that there is some support in the literature for role blurring (Hallett, 1995: 302). However, in her study participants argued that coordination was most effective when individual professionals were clear about their roles and the ways in which they contributed to the overall process of child protection. Most of the professions in her study (general practitioners, psychologists, psychiatrists, lawyers, teachers and accident and emergency doctors) were perceived as having little overlap with other professions. The only major area of overlap seemed to be between social workers and health visitors. Hallett discussed the issue in the following way:

> *It is likely that this [the perceived overlap between the roles of social workers and health visitors] reflects, in part a degree of overlap specifically between social work and health visiting which has been noted elsewhere in the literature .... Nonetheless, in this study, health visitors and their managers articulated clearly the general health promotion role of health visiting and expressed a keen wish not to be involved inappropriately in offering support to families which could, and they argued should, more appropriately be provided by social workers .... However ... the thresholds of intervention and the resource position in social services departments were such that, in practice, health visitors were required to work supportively with families, undertaking similar tasks to social workers.* (Hallett, 1995: 302).

Although coordination may involve joint working, in practice practitioners seem most comfortable when they have clearly defined roles and they can contribute to the overall coordination of services through the effective discharge of their own role. However, to ensure this actually happens requires two further elements: sharing of information, so that practitioners are involved in a case as appropriate; and, in complex cases, a process of joint decision making, so that each practitioner is oriented to a common and shared objective.

Hallett noted that sharing of information is particularly important at crucial points in the decision-making process. In child protection, this exchange of information occurred early on to facilitate decision making about the nature and level of concern:

> *Information exchange was the most prominent form of coordination. It was particularly evident at the referral stage and in initial child protection conferences .... At the referral stages ... there were ready and easy contacts between social services departments and most of the key agencies of which, in this study, schools and health visitors were identified as particularly important.* (Hallett, 1995: 326–7).

The third element identified by Hallett was shared decision making. As she noted, the literature on interprofessional relations stresses the differences and potential conflicts between professions. However, in her study she found very little conflict in the decision-making process. One possible reason for this is the risky nature of child protection decisions and the disastrous consequences of getting child protection decisions wrong:

> *in the context of considerable anxiety of decision-making and fear of the consequences of getting it wrong, tendencies towards consensus and deferring towards those deemed to 'know' are accentuated.* (Hallett, 1995: 331).

As Hallett observed, the joint decision-making process is highly routinised or, in her words, 'circumscribed, bureaucratic and technical' (Hallett, 1995: 330). Since, as we noted in Chapter 2, societal response to failures in child protection tends to be to blame, it is not surprising that no particular profession or individual wishes to stand out against the consensus decision. Furthermore, this area of policy is so important that central government has established dominant objectives and values through legislation. The 1989 Children Act gives precedence and priority to the welfare of vulnerable children over all other objectives and Parton observed that many social workers are almost exclusively concerned 'with the investigation of child abuse and the investigation of risk' (Parton, 1999: 16).

The effective care and support of vulnerable individuals in the community depends on the effective coordination of all the services which are intended to provide them with care and support. However, divisions between agencies providing this support, which have been reinforced by traditional professional rivalries, have meant that some vulnerable clients have fallen into the gaps between agencies with disastrous consequences both for themselves and for others.

This problem has been officially acknowledged since the 1970s and measures were taken to improve the coordination between agencies and the professionals who work for them. These developments have been particularly evident in child protection services and services for individuals with severe mental illness.

HOW TEAMS WORK

In the remainder of this chapter we draw on our ENB-funded research to explore the impact of multidisciplinary work on risk management and decision making. We derive the majority of the data from observation of the operation of nine multidisciplinary teams, six providing services for vulnerable clients in their own homes and three providing services within either a residential or a day care setting. The data presented in this section are derived from field work with each of the teams. During the field work, the researcher interviewed a variety of team members, 'shadowed' at least one community nurse and observed a range of team meetings. This created a rich source of information on different aspects of the teams' work. In the final section we draw on data from the debrief interviews with our diarists to explore in more detail the impact of multidisciplinary practice on risk management.

In this section we start by examining the nature of teamwork and in the following sections we develop the analysis by exploring the impact of teams on the role of nurses and on decision making.

There were both similarities and marked differences between the teams in our study. The obvious common theme was that teamwork brought nurses into regular contact with professionals and practitioners from other disciplines and agencies. However, the precise relationship varied. At one extreme was a residential nursing home managed and staffed by nurses in which practitioners from other disciplines and agencies were used as specialist consultants on a sessional basis or when required (see Box 5.1).

Box 5.1 Team at Elizabeth Nursing Home

Location

Private nursing home registered for 58 people and forming part of a larger complex providing care and support for a variety of vulnerable individuals. The unit provided continuing 24-hour care for frail older people. Some of the clients were self-financing but most were funded by social services.

The team and its operation

The day-to-day care of the residents was provided by the nursing team, led by the matron and deputy matron who were both RGNs, assisted by unqualified support workers. Sessions were provided by a remedial therapist and a physiotherapist. Residents' GPs played an important role in the home: for example, in an emergency the home contacted the GP first rather than taking the resident straight to hospital. All falls were recorded and reported to the appropriate GP.

Box 5.2 The Jubilee Outreach Team

Location

An outreach team based in a day hospital for older people that provided support for older people living at home, aged 75, who had continuing health-care needs.

The team and its operation

The aim of the team was to prevent hospital readmission and promote independence. The team accepted referrals from a number of sources, including hospital ward staff, GPs and from geriatricians following domiciliary visits. The team members included a nurse, an occupational therapist and a physiotherapist and worked closely with the day hospital nurses and geriatric consultants. One of the consultants saw himself as the team leader.

At the other extreme was a small outreach team for older people which was attached to a day hospital (see Box 5.2). Individual members of the team had a clearly defined role. For example, the team nurse illustrated how she saw each of the professional's roles by breaking down an activity of daily living, in this instance, elimination:

> *the physiotherapist would be interested in how the patient was mobilising to the toilet and what equipment they needed to get there; the OT would be interested in equipment around and on the toilet to help make the patient safer, for example hand rails or high toilet seats; and the nurse would be interested in the actual process of elimination, any incontinence, any elimination patterns and whether the patient needed any further investigations.*

The core team members – a nurse, an occupational therapist and a physiotherapist – shared a room in the day hospital and had developed close working relations. This cooperation was reinforced by their practice of making home visits together: as a team they had agreed that it saved time and reduced intrusion into a client's home and the repetition of assessment questions. However, the nurse member also visited clients on her own and during these solo visits she collected information for other team members and health professionals such as the district nurse.

Most other teams involved a variety of professionals, usually health professionals, although occasionally from other sectors such as social workers and care assistants. Generally, as in the Southfield Community Learning

---

Box 5.3 Southfield Community Learning Disability Team

Location

A new multidisciplinary forensic team was established in former NHS premises following the closure of a local learning disability hospital.

The team and its operation

The forensic team provided a secure unit for adults with a learning disability within a secure residential unit. The team on this unit included psychiatrists, psychologists, registered nurses, support workers and therapists. The majority of clients were admitted through the courts, although some clients were admitted informally as emergencies, if they were judged to be a danger to themselves or to the public.

Disability Team, these professionals had clearly defined roles and actual joint working was limited (Box 5.3).

The relationship between team members was relatively unstable; in four of the nine teams we visited, the relationship between team members was under active discussion. For example, Northmount Community Learning Disability Team was actively involved in the closure of a long-stay hospital and it provided a variety of support services. In this team, the community nurses shared premises with social services and other members of the multidisciplinary team. Although the health and social services teams were currently separately managed, they were moving towards integration and joint working. The researcher attended a meeting in which issues of joint working were explored. The meeting was attended by a social services representative, the senior social services manager and two health service managers, the community nurse manager and senior nurse manager. The meeting finalised details such as the name of the team and a launch event. However, there were clearly some unresolved issues. Everyone discussed the precise meaning of the concept of a team and in particular whether core team members had to be interchangeable. They decided to hold a team building day organised by an external facilitator. Among the issues for discussion would be whether occupational therapists and speech therapists should hold clients as a primary worker or acting in an advisory or consultancy role be part of a duty rota. It was clear from the discussion that there were a number of unresolved issues: for example, the nature of the duty system, nurses' roles and where the case notes would be held. No decisions had been made on the management structure for the new team and the senior nurse manager stated that there would have to be some new guidelines for entries in case notes which were in line with UKCC guidance.

ROLE OF NURSES

In most teams, the nurse members' prime role was to provide nursing care and support for service users. Thus, in Hightown Community Mental Health Team, each community psychiatric nurse had a case load of clients and saw his or her clients either at the unit in an individual or a group session, at the client's home or in hospital or the residential unit. They also accompanied clients on outpatient appointments and attended various review meetings with or on behalf of clients.

The Victoria Team for Older People with Memory Impairment was located in a specialist day hospital. The nursing members of the team took overall responsibility for the management and operation of the hospital. Together with support workers they organised the day-to-day general running of the unit: for example, ensuring clients arrived at the start of their session, were ready to leave at the end and received appropriate care and treatment while they were in the unit. The nurses were responsible for administering medicines and any clinical treatments. They ran some of the activity groups, assessing clients and documenting their participation. They attended the doctors' clinics, case conferences, review meetings, home assessment visits and did their own assessments. They often helped to orientate the clients around the building, showing them where to hang their coats and where the toilets were. The unit did not provide a bathing facility and this had caused some difficulties with local fundholding GPs, who sent their clients to cheaper, less-stimulating environments which did provide a bathing facility. The nurses were able to provide family carers and other professionals in the team with information about how the client was functioning in the day hospital. The nurses managed the interface of the unit with other agencies. For example, they had recently had problems with the ambulance crews about collecting clients from the unit. Ambulance crews were arriving at the same time and calling out the clients' names simultaneously. This created confusion and increased clients' anxiety. The nurse manager had agreed a change of practice with the ambulance services. The arrival of the ambulance crews was staggered and unit staff identified the clients and ensured their names were marked on a list before they left.

Overall, the nature of the teams had shaped the role of nurse managers. In many teams not only were they responsible for managing the nurse members of the team but they were also expected to provide support and coordination for the whole team. For example, Eastbridge had been served by a community mental handicap team in the 1980s but with the implementation of the health service and community care reforms the team had broken up and individual learning disability nurses had been attached to general practices. The NHS trust responsible for community health services had reviewed the service and decided to re-establish the team and give the job to a nurse manager. Thus, at the time of the research, the nurse manager was not only responsible for managing all the community learning disability nurses and the staff in the associated residential unit but was also responsible for re-establishing the multidisciplinary team.

In some teams, this expansion of the role of the nurse managers meant that they were engaged in activities that did not fall within the traditional remit of nursing. We shadowed a clinical nurse specialist in Northmount Community Learning Disability Team who was responsible for 20 'tenancies'. When the researcher shadowed him, the early part of his day was spent sorting out staffing problems, trying to avoid using bank [casual] staff because of the expense. He also had to counsel a newly registered staff nurse in charge of one of the houses as he felt that she was still in the student role. He was concerned that she was spending time socialising outside work with the support staff and that the staff were getting too familiar with her and not respecting her. Once he had dealt with his staffing issues, he turned his attention to a major incident. One client had left his home without the agreement of the staff and crossed a busy main road, and as a result the nurse had to investigate and report on the incident. This involved a number of activities:

◆ visiting the house;
◆ reviewing the client's risk assessment;
◆ investigating by interviewing the two staff on duty at the time and taking written statements;
◆ examining ways of preventing a recurrence of the incident;
◆ reporting to his senior manager.

When the clinical nurse specialist returned to his office he had to deal with a range of administrative issues, especially approving the purchase of an item for one of the tenancies. If the team purchased an item for one of the houses which was to be shared and paid for by all tenants, then he had to secure the agreement of the tenants' relatives. For example, if they bought a music centre for three tenants and one died, he felt the relatives could claim a share of the value of the item which had been purchased. There needed to be an agreed way of working out this value. The team had to demonstrate that they were not abusing clients financially.

DECISION MAKING

The nature of decision making which we observed reflected the structure of the teams and the roles of nurses within the team. Since most nurses worked autonomously within the framework of their teams, most of their decisions related to their individual clinical relationship with their clients. However, the broader team did influence this decision making in two ways. Individual nurses were affected by and contributed to team decisions: for example, whom to accept for assessment and/or treatment. In some circumstances individual nurses also needed the resources and expertise of other team members and therefore sought to involve other team members in the assessment of the treatment process.

Individual decision making

Although nurses in our study worked within a team context, in practice they were the 'front-line' staff who had to deal with events as and when they arose. If they visited a client at home and identified a dangerous situation, they had to take immediate action. They might subsequently report their decision and action to other team members.

In Newtown Community Team for the Care of Older People with Mental Health Problems, we shadowed a community mental health nurse. While we were shadowing her she visited an elderly woman who had dementia which left her with a poor short-term memory and limited mobility due to strokes. The nurse identified that the client had a number of risks:

◆ leaving the front door open;
◆ burning food and pans;
◆ going out and money going missing from her home.

The police had been involved and wished to install surveillance equipment, but at the time of the visit a decision on this had not been taken. When she arrived at the house the door was open and the client was distressed, stating that more money had gone and she wanted to die. The nurse made an assessment of the client's mental state, asking her whether she was serious about wanting to die and whether she had any suicidal intentions. She decided that the client was not in immediate danger and there was not a high probability that she would kill herself. She accepted the client's assurances that she would not do anything about taking her own life. However, the nurse was concerned about the client's safety so she took measures to protect her. She:

◆ wrote a message for the home help in the client's communication book to make her aware that this conversation had taken place;
◆ arranged to phone the client later in the day;
◆ offered the client a 'holiday' in a residential home to give her a rest from all the stress of the burglaries.

The client declined the offer of a 'holiday'. The nurse decided that no further action was necessary at this stage.

Sharing information and responsibility

In some circumstances, nurses need rapid access to the expertise and advice of other professionals. This was particularly evident in community mental health teams when clients' conditions changed rapidly and it was difficult to assess whether they would harm themselves or others. Given the uncertainty of the situation, the nurse responsible for the case needed to collect and distribute as much information as possible.

This can be clearly seen in an incident which took place in Lowford Community Mental Health Team. The nurse who we were shadowing was acting as 'duty' nurse in the team office. In the course of a telephone call a distressed client talked about suicide and then 'hung up'. The nurse decided to try to re-establish contact and so phoned back, but the client refused to speak and again terminated the call. The nurse then decided to get more information, so he checked with the client's general practice to see if they had had any recent contact and checked on the availability of the client's key workers. Since the GP had not had any recent contact and both the client's key workers were on holiday, the duty nurse decided to deal with the case himself and phoned the client back. This time the client agreed to talk and the nurse was able to assess the suicide risk and provide 'treatment'. The nurse decided there was no immediate threat of suicide, accepting the client's assurance that he would not take an overdose of tablets, discussed the situation with the client and agreed a coping strategy. Following the call, the duty nurse contacted the GP's surgery, reported the conversation, asked the receptionist to tell the GP and documented the episode in the client's notes.

We observed a similar incident in Hightown Community Mental Health Team. The nurse we were shadowing received a message from a community pharmacist concerning one of her clients. Her client was in a distressed state in the pharmacist's shop and the pharmacist was worried about the client's safety. The client was an informal resident at the bedded unit but had left the night before. The nurse was concerned about this client, because the client was losing weight and not taking her medication. The nurse discussed the situation informally with the psychiatrist and they agreed that the client was in danger and that the nurse should go to the pharmacist's shop and try to bring the client back to the unit so that she could be assessed.

Joint decisions

Most teams have regular team meetings to discuss the general operation of the team and individual clients. Indeed, in some teams, the two activities are combined. For example, the team at Elizabeth Nursing Home had frequent team meetings which were closely modelled on hospital handovers. At each shift change, all available staff met and discussed the events of the past shift and planned the next. The residents were discussed and issues that affected specific residents identified: for example, if a resident was not eating or needed a change to a wound dressing. Any planned events were noted, such as hospital outpatient appointments or review meetings.

In most teams, the two functions were separated. High Town Community Mental Health Team held a weekly meeting to discuss team issues. This meeting did include the allocation of any new clients, but the detailed discussion of clients took place in separate individual review meetings.

Meetings about individual clients were generally seen as the most important type of joint meeting. In the Jubilee Outreach Team there were two types of client-oriented meetings: informal meetings between core team members and more formal review meetings which also included the medical consultants. Since the core team members shared an office, they had regular informal meetings in which they shared information about clients and discussed actions and assessments. For example, at one such meeting the physiotherapist asked the nurse if she could look at a client's leg ulcers as she felt that they were deteriorating. In contrast, the weekly review meetings were more structured and were led by the consultants. Two such review meetings observed by the researcher followed the same format. The consultant had the medical notes and used these to provide details of names, diagnoses and medication. The other team members provided information from assessments and visits. The consultant used this information to make decisions, such as discharges from the team, entry to the day hospital and outpatient follow up.

The structure and degree of formalisation of client-oriented meetings in teams tended to vary according to the level of participation of users and their carers. The involvement of service users and/or carers tended to formalise meetings; at a minimum, there had to be a set time and an agenda. For example, in Victoria Day Hospital for People with Memory Impairment, users and carers were invited to a meeting that reviewed the user's progress. We attended a review meeting chaired by a community mental health nurse. The meeting was attended by a G grade nurse from the day hospital, a social worker, a social services care manager, a representative from the care-providing agency and the client's family. The mental health nurse stated that the aim was to discuss what had happened since the last review. The first part of the meeting considered the client's current care. The day hospital nurse described how the client functioned: she had a high level of attendance, enjoyed herself there and there were no management problems with her. The carer's family described the management problems they were experiencing at home. Her poor memory meant that she was disorientated and wandered, and was therefore putting herself at risk. She was unsafe in the kitchen. The social worker discussed the findings of the Community Care Assessment and concluded that the client needed the protection of 24-hour care. The second part of the meeting addressed the future. The family reluctantly agreed that the client should go into residential care and the meeting discussed the practicalities of the move.

By contrast, the involvement of users was particularly well developed in learning disability and mental health services. In the Southfield Community Learning Disability Team a care plan meeting for each client was held at regular intervals which they were invited to attend and discuss their progress and any problems. The care planning meetings were designed to monitor progress with the care, to identify any new problems and set new goals. One meeting we attended included the client, the speech and language therapist, the unit staff nurse and the occupational therapist. There did not appear to be a formal chairperson. There was no medical input at this meeting. The client, whose care plan was reviewed, had recently absconded. During the meeting the client became upset and the meeting explored the reasons for this. The client was upset about three specific issues:

◆ not sleeping well despite reports to the contrary by the night staff;
◆ not having enough time with his key worker;
◆ coming off a Section of the Mental Health Act and being discharged into the community.

Once the client's concerns had been identified, the speech therapist took control of the meeting and a plan of action was agreed. The implementation of the agreed plan was mainly delegated to the staff nurse.

In the community, individual nursing practice and decision making tend to be embedded within multidisciplinary teams. The individual nurse needs the support of the team to deal with crises and complex cases. Team decisions, especially about the management of individual cases, provide the context for individual practice.

The balance of individual and joint decision making

In this section we have argued that individual nurses are involved both in individual decision making when they work with clients on a one-to-one basis and joint decisions, especially when they participate in team meetings. To show how these are linked together we concentrate on the activities of one experienced community mental health nurse, who we refer to as Sally, who worked in a well-established community mental health team and had an active case load of 26 clients, some of whom she saw weekly. We observed her activities over a 4-day period and we concentrate on a single day which she felt was fairly typical.

Box 5.4 Summary of an experienced community mental health nurse's activities

9.00–9.25	Prepares for day's work; information exchange with colleagues; phone calls from clients; prioritising work.
9.30–10.00	Attends team meeting, receives information and participates in discussion.
10.05–10.40	Visits self-harming client A to assess mood and advise on discharge from section of the Mental Health Act. Client A is at home on leave from residential unit.
10.50–11.00	Visits residential unit to give her assessment of client A.
11.05–12.10	Attends meeting at resource centre to negotiate move of five clients from under-65 team to over-65 team.
12.15–1.00	Interviews and assesses client B with eating disorder.
1.00–2.00	Eats lunch and writes reports about clients visited.
2.05–2.55	Collects client C and takes him to an appointment with his GP; on return journey, questions client about appointment.
3.00–3.55	Collects client D and takes him to an appointment with his GP; on return journey, questions client about appointment.
4.05–4.40	Interviews client E, self-harming mother with eating disorder; decides to consult specialist therapy team and child protection team.
4.50–5.15	Writes up notes and completes paper work.

During this day the nurse spent the majority of her time visiting and working with individual clients (see Box 5.4). When she spent time with her clients she was assessing their condition and making decisions about their future treatment even if the overt purpose of their interaction was different. For example, after her lunch, Sally spent 2 hours collecting clients and taking them to their GP appointments. The overt purpose of this meeting was to ensure that they attended their appointments with the GP who could then monitor their treatment, especially their medication. However, Sally used the journey to collect information. For example, she asked client C what had happened when he saw the doctor and he commented that the GP wanted to give him more pills but he didn't want them because 'they muck up your liver'. Afterwards Sally told the researcher that she felt client C was in good form, as his speech was clear and he was in good humour, so she had decided not to see him for 6 weeks.

Although Sally worked with her clients on a one-to-one basis, in some cases her assessments formed part of a more complex decision-making process. For example, her morning visit to client A was explicitly linked to a multiprofessional meeting. Client A had a history of self-harm, including one serious suicide attempt, and was currently undergoing compulsory treatment in a residential unit. He was at home on weekend leave and Sally was assessing his condition to see if she felt he was ready to be discharged. Following the assessment, she went to the unit to report on and write up her assessment. The following day she attended the discharge meeting and gave her assessment that the client's condition had improved but there was still cause for concern and she agreed to monitor the client when he was discharged.

In some cases Sally's assessment of a client's condition resulted in a decision to involve other professionals. For example, the last client she saw, client E, had originally been referred to the team as a possible case of postnatal depression. However, the client's mental state deteriorated and she had developed an eating disorder as well as self-harming behaviour. Sally had accepted the client onto her case load and was seeing her twice a week. However, because of lack of progress, she had asked a psychologist to work jointly with her and, indeed, was willing to hand over the case as she did not feel she had any special expertise in this area. She had decided to ask the special therapy team for advice on the management of this client and following her afternoon meeting decided to consult the local child protection team. She did not feel that the woman was likely to harm her child but she wanted to contact the team for advice and support.

Sally also attended two meetings; the first was a team meeting in which the team leader provided information about various recent developments in agency policy and identified issues that the team needed to address – for example, the consequences of his own departure and how they would deal with a client who refused to see anyone except him. The second meeting involved a negotiation between two teams over the transfer of clients. Sally attended as a representative of the under-65 team who were seeking to persuade the over-65 team to take four of their clients. Sally was able to negotiate a phased transfer of the clients with a handover period so that the nurses in the over-65 team could get to know the clients and their management. In particular, Sally agreed to arrange a session to demonstrate the techniques associated with depot injections that formed part of the treatment regime of several of the clients, as the nurses in the over-65s team considered themselves to be out of practice with injections.

It is clear from this account that although Sally was responsible for managing her own case load, and primarily did this through the medium of one-to-one sessions, the assessments and decisions which she took within these sessions were linked to the broader context of the team in number of ways. The overall allocation of work both within and between teams had to be negotiated and agreed. Sally collected information for and participated in meetings that made significant decisions about individual clients, for example discharge meetings. Sally used some client interviews as opportunities not only to monitor their mental state and to decide whether she needed to involve other professionals in the client's management but also to obtain information about their interaction with other professionals, for example, their general practitioner.

COMMENT

Most nurses in our study worked as part of a team, often a multiprofessional team. These teams provided the framework within which they undertook their nursing practice. We identified two levels of decision making, individual and team decisions. The majority of nurses' time was taken up with providing direct care and support for individual service users, often in one-to-one meetings. Within these meetings individual nurses assessed users and made decisions about their treatment. Much of this work was seen as relatively routine and therefore did not require wider involvement or participation. The nurse could choose how and in what way to make the decision, usually relying on his or her own judgement. However, some decisions involved wider team participation, either because the nurse did not feel he or she had the expertise, or because of the high consequence if anything went wrong or because it involved resources that the individual practitioner did not have. In this case the nurse was involved in wider decision making, sometimes by the whole team. The precise role of the nurse depended on the significance of the decision for her particular client. If a team decision affected his or her client, then the nurse was actively involved, especially in providing information about his or her client's physical and mental state. However, if the decision did not affect their clients directly, then nurses tended to play a more passive role. They were often happy to play this role, leaving the active role to other participants, such as nurse managers.

6

Improving the quality of risk management and decision making in practice

Andy Alaszewski   *Helen Alaszewski*

INTRODUCTION

In Chapters 4 and 5 we explored the ways in which nurses manage risk and make decisions both individually and as part of a multiprofessional team. In this chapter we explore the ways in which nurses are taught and learn to manage risk. We start with a discussion of the literature and then relate the findings of our ENB-funded research to current approaches.

DEVELOPING COMPETENCE IN RISK MANAGEMENT AND DECISION MAKING

We begin our analysis with a general discussion of the aims of nurse education, which are to prepare the 'competent' nurse. We then consider the importance of risk management as an aspect of competence.

Competence in nursing

Central to the professional training is the development of the competent practitioner who is 'adequately qualified for a task' (Sykes, 1982: 192). However, the precise definition of the competent practitioner is elusive. As Duffield (1991: 59) argued, competence 'requires a fit between a role, the scope of practice and the individual's skills for the job'. Thus, the skills of the competent practitioner are appropriate and sufficient for the tasks which fall within his or her scope of practice.

The nature of competence depends on the nature of the task or role: thus, for a 'craft' such as pottery or driving a car, the competent practitioner must have appropriate practical skills. The assessment of this type of competence is based mainly on the assessment of practical skills, either in the craftsman's 'masterpiece' or in a driving test. The competent nurse is expected not only to have appropriate skills but also to have the theoretical knowledge which enables him or her to understand whether the application of a particular skill is appropriate and what the likely effects of its application will be. As Lankshear *et al.* (1996) pointed out in their discussion of nursing, although there is no agreed definition of the concept of competency, most definitions include reference to appropriate knowledge and appropriate skills for a particular task or job. This can be seen in the 'statements' of competence which underpin vocational qualifications. These statements are designed to 'be relevant to work' and 'facilitate entry into, or progression in employment' (Fletcher, 1991: 19) and should include certain specifications (Box 6.1).

However, the competence of modern professionals includes not only appropriate skills and supporting knowledge but also appropriate values. Parsons in his classic study of the medical profession, drew attention to 'the complexity and subtlety of the knowledge and skill and the consequent length and intensity of training' (Parsons, 1951: 434) required to produce the competent doctor.

Within nursing, values tend to be discussed in terms of appropriate 'attitudes'. For example, Duffield noted that the term 'skill' is often used interchangeably with competencies, but she argued that competencies should:

> *signify not only the performance of a task, but also the underlying knowledge and attitudes to practice or perform the task.* (Duffield, 1991: 56).

Box 6.1 Statement of competence (Fletcher, 1991: 19)

◆ Skills to specified standards.

◆ Relevant knowledge and understanding.

◆ The ability to use and apply knowledge.

◆ Understanding to the performance of relevant tasks.

The framework for defining and assessing the competence of nurses, who are eligible for registration by the national body for nursing, the United Kingdom Council for Nursing, Midwives and Health Visitors, is established by law and is generally referred to as Rule 18 (Box 6.2).

Box 6.2 Rule 18

(2) The Common Foundation Programme and the Branch Programme shall be designed to prepare the student to assume the responsibilities and accountability that registration confers and to prepare the nursing student to apply knowledge and skills to meet the nursing needs of individuals and of groups in health and in sickness in the area of practice of the Branch Programme and shall include enabling the student to achieve the following outcomes:

(a) the identification of the social and health implications of pregnancy and child bearing, physical and mental handicap, disease, disability or ageing for the individual, her or his friends, family and community;

(b) the recognition of common factors which contribute to, and those which adversely affect, physical, mental and social well-being of patients and clients and take appropriate action;

(c) the use of relevant literature and research to inform the practice of nursing;

(d) the appreciation of the influence of social, political and cultural factors in relation to health care;

(e) an understanding of the requirements of legislation relevant to the practice of nursing;

(f) the use of appropriate communication skills to enable the development of helpful caring relationships with patients and clients and their families and friends, and to initiate and conduct therapeutic relationships with patients and clients;

(g) the identification of health-related learning needs of patients and clients, families and friends to participate in health promotion;

(h) an understanding of the ethics of health care and of the nursing profession and the responsibilities which these impose on the nurse's professional practice;

(i) the identification of the needs of the patients and clients to enable them to progress from varying degrees of dependence to maximum independence, or to a peaceful death;

(j) the identification of physical, psychological, social and spiritual needs of the patient or clients; an awareness of values and concepts of individual care, the ability to devise a plan of care, contribute to its implementation and evaluation and the demonstration of the application of the principles of a problem-solving approach to the practice of nursing;

> **Box 6.2** Cont'd
>
> (k) the ability to function effectively in a team and participate in a multi-professional approach to the care of patients and clients;
>
> (l) the use of the appropriate channel of referral for matters not within her sphere of competence;
>
> (m) the assignment of appropriate duties to others and the supervision, teaching and monitoring of assigned duties.
>
> *The Nurses, Midwives and Health Visitors (Registered Fever Nurses Amendment Rules and Training Amendment Rules) Approval Order* (1989) No 1456.

There is no direct equivalent to Rule 18 for post-registration training but the English National Board does provide outline curricula for its various awards. These tend to refer to the extension of the competence of the registered nurse but avoid defining this extension. For example, one of the courses in our survey, a post-registration course for nurses working with individuals with learning disabilities, included the following statement of aims:

> *To extend the competence of the registered nurse for the Mentally Handicapped through education and experience to further their skills as practitioners within the context of a multi-agency service making appropriate nursing interventions and giving support to people with mental handicap.*

Although Rule 18 and the various outline curricula provide the general framework for competence, there is no consensus within nurse education on the best way to operationalise the concept. Two contrasted approaches have developed, the empirical and the ideological.

The dominant empirical approach concentrates on identifying the specific skills which contribute to the overall development of competence. These specific components are identified either by observing practitioners (see Benner's (1984) comparison of practitioners at different stages in their development) or more commonly by seeking a consensus view within areas of practice (see Lankshear *et al.* (1996) for an analysis of competencies in a number of nurse specialisms). This approach to identifying competence tends to fragment the concepts into a range of specialist skills. For example, Lankshear and her colleagues identified 106 skills in their 'map' of competence for mental health nursing (Lankshear *et al.*, 1996: 144–9).

The alternative approach emphasises the underlying ideology. It involves identifying the main objectives which practice is designed to achieve and then examining the ways in which practitioners can contribute to the achievement of these objectives. We refer to it as ideological as it often starts from a strong ideological position which is used to define the purpose of practice. Brooker and his colleagues used it in their study of the educational preparation of nurses for working with older people. Using ageism (the stereotyping of older people as incompetent and dependent) as a starting point their study was designed:

> *to determine the extent to which pre- and post-registration educational programmes in nursing in England prepare practitioners to promote patient/client autonomy in the provision of the care to older people, including frail older people.* (Brooker *et al.*, 1997: 9).

This 'gold standard' is then used to assess the competence of actual practitioners and, in particular, the extent to which they fall short of ideal standards. For example, the findings of one part of the research were summarised in the following way:

> *Observation of thirty nurses in a range of care settings and ratings of care events revealed wide variations in the extent to which individual nurses demonstrate an awareness of strategies for promoting autonomy and independence within their practice. While most nurses incorporate some degree of information-giving and attempts to gain feedback into their day-to-day practice with older people, they appear to be less skilled at involving patients and clients in decisions about their plan of care.* (ENB, 1997: p. 3).

Risk and nursing competence

Despite the differences between these two studies, both identified risk assessment and management as important elements of the 'competent' nurse. Lankshear and her colleagues identified it both in general and mental health nursing but gave it particular prominence in mental health nursing (Box 6.3).

Box 6.3 Risk assessment and management in mental health nursing (Lankshear *et al.*, 1996: 166)

The qualitative section of the report highlights the '... considerable interest in developing skills related to increasing the predictive validity of such [risk] assessments' ... The results of the survey suggest that mental health nurses all recognise the growing importance of this element of the nurse's role in the future. There were four 'risk assessment' competencies included in the survey.

4.1 Making and acting upon decisions which carry risks to patients/clients
4.2 Making and acting upon decisions which carry risks to families
4.3 Making and acting upon decisions which carry risks to communities
4.4 Making and acting upon decisions which carry risks to the organisation

Each of these saw their relative importance rise considerably with, for example, 68% of respondents seeing 4.1 as important for their future role.

Brooker and his colleagues identified risk, especially concerns with safety, as a potential impediment to enhancing the independence and autonomy of older people:

> *Universally high scores in relation to the promotion of patient safety suggest that nurses may find it difficult to determine an appropriate degree of risk and … may unwittingly be threatening the personal autonomy of older patients and clients as a consequence. This finding reflects the analysis of course curricula in Phase I of the study which suggested that the issues of patient participation and risk-taking are insufficiently covered within most programmes.* (Brooker *et al.*, 1997: 184).

Competence is clearly central to the nature of contemporary professional practice. It is a complex concept, involving appropriate skills, knowledge and attitudes, and different approaches will tend to emphasise different aspects. Within nursing, Rule 18 provides a legal framework for defining nursing competence. Although risk is not mentioned in Rule 18, it is clearly implicit within it.

DEVELOPING COMPETENCE: RATIONAL ANALYSIS OR REFLECTIVE PRACTICE

In this section we consider approaches to risk education in nursing. The first approach builds on the 'skills' approach to competence and seeks to identify and enhance specific skills in risk management and decision making through formal teaching, especially through the explicit use of decision-support technologies. The second approach builds on the 'ideological' approach to competence and seeks to provide nurses with greater understanding, insight and skills and through doing this can be seen as a way of enhancing their ability to manage risk and make decisions.

Formal teaching about risk and decision making

Within health care, there is a well-established tradition of formal education which relies on the use of decision-support technologies that are designed to help the individual professional understand the decision-making process and make better decisions. Advocates of the use of decision-support technologies argue that the behaviour of decision makers can be classified along a cognitive continuum – at one end of the continuum is intuition and at the other end is analysis:

> *Intuitive thought involves rapid, unconscious data processing that combines the available information by 'averaging' it, has low consistency, and is*

moderately accurate .... Analysis, the other end of the cognitive continuum, has the opposite effect. Analytic thought is slow, conscious, and consistent; it is usually quite accurate (though it occasionally produces large errors); and it is quite likely to combine information, using organizing principles that are more complicated than simple 'averaging'. (Hamm, 1988: 82–3).

Decision-support technologies seek to move decision making along the cognitive continuum by formalising and making explicit the assumptions being made by the decision maker. Although, as Dowie pointed out, such changes may not necessarily improve the quality of decision making, it should make them more transparent, 'a criterion mandatory for public decisions of all kinds' (Dowie, 1999: 43).

The application of decision-support technologies to medical decision making has been well documented. For example, Dowie and Elstein (1988b) in their collection of material on clinical decision making included three case studies. All three cases illustrated this approach using doctors' decisions made within a clinical setting. Doubilet and McNeil (1988) used acute appendicitis and carotoid endarterectomy, Klein and Pauker (1988) the treatment of recurrent deep vein thrombosis in pregnancy and Elstein *et al.* (1988) oestrogen replacement for menopausal women. As we discussed at the end of Chapter 4, Dowie (1999) developed this work and provided a general framework which can be applied to nursing decision making. He constructed a way of separating out the technical components of decision making, such as assessments of probabilities, from the value issues, such as assessments of utilities.

The 'skills-based' approach to developing competence in risk management and decision making involves the use of explicit teaching of decision making and risk management strategies. These could be taught in class but the emphasis would be on using 'real' examples and then reinforcing the skills through actual use in practice settings.

Reflective practice

The 'skills' approach is designed to enhance the technical ability of nurses to manage risk and make decisions; however, it does not necessarily ensure that the decisions are sensitive to the specific circumstance of each case. Clinical decisions are made in relationship to specific individuals. They relate to the unique characteristics of each case and often involve issues of values, especially when there is tension between different interests in the decision-making process. More 'general' technical knowledge will not necessarily assist with the unique case and it will certainly not resolve conflicts of values.

The rational approach to decision making can be seen as a threat to professional autonomy and judgement. A mechanistic approach to risk and

decision making threatens to turn professionals into rule-following bureau-
crats, and there is a danger that, in rejecting this approach, individual
practitioners will see the only alternative as rule breaking. As we mentioned
earlier, Schön has identified an alternative approach which does not seek to
externalise decision making through a decision-making support system but
seeks to enhance the decision-making skills of the individual through a
process of reflection. Schön argued that professionals deal with uncertainty,
which often cannot be reduced through technical rationality, for example,
through the collection and use of more evidence or information:

> *In real-world practice, problems do not present themselves to the*
> *practitioner as givens. They must be constructed from the materials of*
> *problematic situations which are puzzling, troubling, and uncertain. In*
> *order to convert a problematic situation to a problem, a practitioner must*
> *do a certain kind of work. He must make sense of an uncertain situation*
> *that initially makes no sense. When professionals consider what road to*
> *build, for example, they deal usually with a complex and ill-defined*
> *situation in which geographic, topological, financial, economic, and*
> *political issues are all mixed up together. Once they have somehow decided*
> *what road to build and go on to consider how best to build it, they may*
> *have a problem they can solve by the application of available techniques;*
> *but when the road they have built leads unexpectedly to the destruction of a*
> *neighbourhood, they may find themselves again in a situation of*
> *uncertainty.* (Schön, 1988: 66–7).

Schön argued that the individual practitioner needs to respond to the unique
characteristics of a specific case through a systematic process of reflection so
that he or she both seeks to identify the nature of the problem and its best
solution:

> *When a practitioner reflects in and on his practice, the possible objects of*
> *his reflection are as varied as the kinds of phenomena before him and the*
> *systems of knowing-in-practice which he brings to them. He may reflect on*
> *the tacit norms and appreciation which underlie a judgment, or on the*
> *strategies and theories implicit in a pattern of behavior .... When the*
> *phenomenon at hand eludes the ordinary categories of knowledge-in-*
> *practice, presenting itself as unique or unstable, the practitioner may surface*
> *and criticize his initial understanding of the phenomenon, construct a new*
> *description of it, and test the new description by an on-the-spot experiment.*
> *Sometimes he arrives at a new theory of the phenomenon by articulating a*
> *feeling he has about it.* (Schön, 1988: 72).

The education and development of the 'reflective' practitioner needs to
start with and from the reality of everyday practice. Reflection needs to

be grounded in practice. Although it is a highly personal process, it can be formalised. This can be done by 'capturing' situations in a reflective diary and analysing them with the assistance of an experienced practitioner or peers.

FORMAL EDUCATION ON RISK AND DECISION MAKING

Curriculum content

Formal education on risk and decision making is conspicuous by its absence in the current nursing curriculum. We undertook a purposive sample of 12 registration and 12 post-registration nurse education programmes in England and found little evidence of systematic formal education in risk management. Eleven courses, including eight post-registration courses, made no explicit reference to risk, either in the overall aims of the course or within the specific content and learning outcomes of individual modules. Even when risk was specifically identified, it tended to form isolated elements within one or more units or modules (see Table 6.1). In a small minority of courses, three registration courses and two post-registration courses, risk did feature more

Table 6.1 Risk-related content of courses

Course	Risk	Location	Theme
01. Diploma Adult Branch	Yes	Unit theme	1. Health promotion (Risk/strategies)
02. Diploma Mental Health	Yes	Unit themes	1. Advocacy 2. Ethical dilemmas 3. Health promotion 4. Risk taking 5. Vulnerability 6. Abuse
03. Diploma Learning Disabilities	Yes	Unit themes	1. Health promotion (risk/strategies) 2. Advocacy/empowerment
04. Diploma Adult Branch			
0.5 Diploma Mental Health	Yes	Indicative content	1. Advocacy 2. Risk taking 3. Risk of dependency
0.6 Diploma Learning Disabilities	Yes	Various	1. Risk awareness 2. Balance, dilemma 3. Empowerment, advocacy 4. Abuse 5. Assessment 6. Risk taking

Table 6.1 Cont'd

Course	Risk	Location	Theme
07. BSc Adult Health	Yes	Module theme	1. Infection control (risk assessment)
08. BSc Mental Health			
09. BSc Adult Health	Yes	Module themes	1. Lifting and handling (risk assessment) 2. Client advocacy 3. Protection from harm
10. BSc Mental Health	Yes	Module themes	1. Empowerment 2. Risk factors in mental health 3. Risk assessment 4. Risk taking
11. BSc Learning Disabilities	Yes	Unit of competence	1. Assessing risk 2. Minimise risk and promote independence 3. Risk management 4. Decision making
12. BSc Learning Disabilities			
13. ENB Elderly	Yes	Unit theme	1. Risk in caring for older people 2. Identifying risk factors 3. Client rights 4. Empowerment
14. ENB Learning Disabilities			
15. ENB Learning Disabilities			
16. ENB Mental Health			
17. ENB Mental Health			
18. ENB Elderly	Yes	Outline syllabus and module aims	1. Advocacy and empowerment 2. Pressure sores (risk assessment) 3. Elder abuse
19. Diploma Learning Disabilities			
20. BA Mental Health	Yes	Risk module plus material in other module	1. Assessment 2. Advocacy and empowerment 3. Vulnerability
21. BSc District Nursing			
22. BSc Learning Disabilities			
23. Diploma Mental Health	Yes		1. Risk assessment
24. MSc Elderly			

prominently but even in these courses there was little evidence of the use of formal approaches to teaching, such as decision-support methodologies.

In three registration courses and two post-registration courses, risk formed a more prominent feature of the curriculum. In one learning disability degree course, whose successful completion conferred professional qualification in both nursing and social work, risk was one of 12 'units of competence'. The documentation is interesting because it identifies outcomes but provides no real information on how these outcomes are actually achieved and, in particular, there appears to be no formal development of skills in risk management or decision making.

The course documentation identified the necessary professional skills. It linked these skills to specific nursing (UKCC) and social work competences (Box 6.4).

The documentation contained a clear statement of the nature and importance of risk management within professional practice:

> The management of risk   *The management of risk is an important*
> *component of the care .... Levels of risk management range from*
> *maintaining a safe environment for self and others, to assessing and*
> *appraising the presence of risk indicators in the course of work with*
> *individuals in the context of their families and/or social networks; devising*

Box 6.4 Curriculum content of a joint course

Relevant UKCC competences

◆ Human rights.
◆ Codes of practice.
◆ Representation and advocacy.
◆ Moral and ethical issues.
◆ Models of promoting health and maximising independence.
◆ Prevention of accidents and first aid.

Relevant social work competences

◆ Ethical issues and dilemmas in practice, including the potential for conflict between organisational, professional and individual values.
◆ Appraise the presence of risk indicators.
◆ Assist in the assessment of individuals deemed at risk under statute and demonstrate a working knowledge of relevant legal issues and administration.
◆ Assess needs, strengths, situations and risks.
◆ Act as an advocate.

Box 6.5 Risk-related learning outcomes for level 3 training

Competent level 3 student:

◆ plans and implements interventions, based on an assessment of risk, to minimise risk and promote independence, with minimum supervision;

◆ uses a structured problem-solving approach to risk management when planning and implementing interventions, with minimum supervision;

◆ takes responsibility for decisions involving risk, with minimum supervision;

◆ when planning interventions, works within legal requirements, policies and procedures, with minimum supervision;

◆ acts upon identified risks which are not addressed adequately by existing services and support networks, with minimum supervision;

◆ when planning and implementing interventions, takes into account perception of risk by client (and family), in relation to linguistic, cultural and religious background, with minimum supervision.

care management plans on the basis of the assessment of risk, and evaluating interventions; managing risk within a legal and ethical framework, and understanding the professional roles within different organisational settings.

The documentation also included specific risk-related learning outcomes for each level of training (Box 6.5).

The documentation did identify issues which students should address but did not specify a formal way in which the students would acquire the appropriate skills (Box 6.6).

Within a post-registration mental health degree programme there was also a risk module that included risk within its aims, content and learning outcomes but it was not evident that formal risk management and decision support systems were used (Box 6.7).

Formal risk teaching

As part of our study we interviewed lecturers, practice teachers and students from each of the 24 courses (a total of 72 interviews). Our interviews with course participants confirmed our analysis of course documentation. Only 18 (25%) sets of respondents felt that risk was formally taught on their course. Actually more students (8, 33%) than course lecturers felt that there was formal class risk teaching (7, 29%).

Some course lecturers sought to justify the lack of formal teaching on their course by asserting that such teaching might 'frighten' students and make

Box 6.6 Assessing risk in a range of settings, with different groups

◆ Least restricted environment.

◆ Balance between dependence/independence (strength/needs).

◆ Medication.

◆ Health and safety in the physical environment (including travel, shopping, cooking for people with learning difficulties).

◆ Ability to build a structured safety-net – issues of professional accountability – problem-solving if safety-net fails.

◆ Sexual vulnerability.

◆ Medical vulnerability.

◆ Physical abuse.

◆ Emotional abuse.

◆ Assessment of service support in the context of risk (policies and procedures – level of support, length of time, pacing).

Box 6.7 Risk assessment within the Care Programme Approach

Aim of module

To develop the skills required to engage in effective risk assessment for all client groups within the framework of the Care Programme Approach.

Synopsis of module

The module will enable development of assessment skills appropriate for both the initial assessment of client risk (including serious risk) and also subsequent risk assessment of those already cared for within the CPA.

Learning outcomes

This module will enable the student to:

◆ Consider the nature of risk as identified within the Care Programme Approach as it applies to specific client groups in different contexts.

◆ Identify factors contributing to risk and examine a range of assessment techniques and practices.

◆ Recognise and discuss the legal and ethical issues surrounding risk assessment.

Box 6.7 Cont'd

Outcome 3

◆ suicide

◆ parasuicide or serious violence

◆ severe self-neglect

◆ violence and neglect from others

◆ risk in different contexts.

Outcome 4

◆ psychiatric, psychological, physical and social factors

◆ risk assessment tools

◆ risk assessment techniques and methodologies.

Outcome 5

◆ client rights and professional responsibility

◆ UKCC Code of Professional Conduct

◆ professional control and civil liberty

◆ statutory obligations and personal ethics.

---

them overanxious. For example, one lecturer on a mental health diploma branch programme put forward an argument about the difficulties of making risk too explicit and the possibility of this leading to students becoming defensive in their practice:

> *I do believe you have to take therapeutic risks, because I believe that's what you do with children all the time. You've got to let them go at some point but how do you do that within a structure which has such a hold or so many potential things that can frighten you or you think I'll get in to trouble if I do this, there's procedure, there's policy. There's the code – I know why it's there and I know it's got to be there and we have to have standards and some kind of framework, but as soon as you do that you're immediately putting constraints on somebody's creativity and ability.*

It is interesting to note that in some courses which did have explicit risk teaching, lecturers were concerned that such teaching could be 'ghettoised' and the students would not make the links between this part of the course and other aspects of teaching and learning. For example, a course lecturer for a learning disability registration course which had a risk module felt that the existence of the module effectively isolated risk teaching from other aspects of the curriculum:

It's (teaching on risk) stuck on. There is not a thread of risk in the curriculum. From the Learning Disability point of view it has its own place, focus and slot on the timetable .... No more than four academic days (out of 340) are devoted to risk teaching.

Risk learning

Most lecturers felt that students learned about risk in college through formal teaching. Not a single mentor felt that students learned about risk in formal teaching sessions. Students were in between: approximately half cited reflection in class as a source of learning but only a third cited formal teaching. In the 72 interviews, there were 431 references to risk learning. When compared to references to teaching there were comparatively fewer references to learning from formal teaching in college (33, 8%).

While both mentors and students played down formal teaching in class, lecturers saw it as an important source of learning about risk. For example, a lecturer on a post-registration learning disability degree course described learning from formal teaching and assessment:

This morning's lecture we've been looking at positive and negative reinforcement and issues surrounding that; I mean it's come to light how often we're not reinforced for the good things that we do. I think if, certainly in assignments, there was a good analysis of a person's situation that reflected on issues of risk we considered it from all points of view; for instance, the one for road safety last year was brilliant.

Some students did recognise formal class teaching as a source of risk learning but usually as an adjunct to other means of learning. For example, a student on a post-registration mental health degree who had completed a risk module commented in the following way:

Researcher:	How do you learn about risk?
Student:	I've obviously been lucky enough to do a course but I would say prior to this you learnt by experience.
Researcher:	You've ... mentioned judgement – how do you think you gain judgement?
Student:	Through experience and through a certain amount of teaching – you do learn things through other subjects about what some of the risk factors might be – being single, alone, having a history of major mental illness – you do learn that there are certain things which would make someone more vulnerable to risk than others. Experimental learning of the factors that make people vulnerable to risk.

In our study of nurse education courses there was little evidence of formal teaching of risk and no evidence of the use of structured decision analysis. Given concerns about professional competence in decision making and risk management, it is difficult to explain this lack of formal instruction. There are some aspects of risk and decision making that are both complex and difficult to understand. Formal teaching could play an important part in preparing students in these areas and enhancing their learning opportunities (see, for example, Stanley and Manthorpe, 1997).

REFLECTIVE PRACTICE, RISK AND DECISION MAKING

Although a minority of respondents in our survey argued that there was formal risk teaching in class, only 13 (18%) of respondents felt that risk was not taught at all. The majority (41, 57%) of respondents felt that risk formed an implicit theme within their course (see Table 6.2). This response was particularly evident amongst course lecturers who frequently argued that risk teaching permeated the curriculum and was implicit rather than explicit.

When invited to assess the amount of time devoted to risk, most of the lecturers were unable to estimate what percentage of curriculum time was devoted to risk or even to identify the particular units within which it was taught. In courses that did not have a risk module, lecturers tended to give vague answers when invited, such as 'a significant amount of time' was spent on issues related to risk. Since it permeated the curriculum it informed all aspects of teaching. One lecturer in a pre-registration diploma adult branch course described how risk fitted into the curriculum in this way:

Table 6.2 Views of risk teaching (values in per cent)

	Explicit	Implicit	Not taught
All *n* = 72	25	56	19
Registration *n* = 36	25	61	14
Post-registration *n* = 36	25	50	25
Lecturers *n* = 24	29	71	
Mentors *n* = 24	13	58	29
Students *n* = 24	33	46	29

I don't know that it fits in as a specific subject, I think it's addressed in individual contexts when we're discussing .... I don't think those ideas are ever brought together under an umbrella heading of risk.

This view, that risk 'crops up' as part of discussion of other topics, was shared by another adult branch lecturer:

It threads all the way through; you wouldn't be able to find a unit on risk. I think we should write one but I think it's too important to restrict to one area of the curriculum so it begins from day one all the way through because safety is very important.

This apparent contradiction can be resolved if we see reflective practice as a form of risk teaching. The overwhelming majority of course documents explicitly referred to reflective practice (see Table 6.3).

Table 6.3 Forms of related-risk teaching and learning

Course	Reflection
Pre-registration	
1	Critical incident analysis
2	Critical incident analysis
3	Critical incident analysis and self-reflection
4	—
5	Development of reflective practice
6	Learning contracts–diaries
7	Learning journals and critical incident analysis
8	Learning contracts and supervision
9	Critical incident analysis and professional development
10	Critical incident analysis and professional development
11	Logs and diaries
12	Learning contracts
Post-registration	
13	Assessment and diary
14	Structured reflection
15	Critical incident analysis and reflective journal
16	Reflective diary
17	Reflective practice and diary
18	Reflective journal
19	Reflective journal
20	Evidence of critical reflection
21	Development of reflective practitioner
22	—
23	Reflective chronicle
24	Critical incident analysis

This type of teaching and learning involved a process of bringing incidents and events into a class room situation either through role play or students' recollection of incidents or events which they recorded in diaries or journals. This approach was well developed in registration courses. For example, in a learning disability degree course there was a clear philosophical commitment to reflective practice which was linked to specific aspects of the curriculum:

The school has a philosophy based on the concept of the reflective practitioner, who engages in continual reflection upon practice, bases his/her practice on current theoretical perspectives, and modifies and extends that theory and practice link by further reflection ....

The strengthening of links [between theory and practice] will be achieved by:

❖ *Introduction to reflective techniques, with the students being made aware of their contribution to the course in the unit: Personal Resource Management.*

❖ *The use of instruments to aid 'reflection-in-action' and 'on-action', for example by the use of learning logs and diaries to record experiences and feelings. Tutorials will be organised to assess what has been experienced and future learning and action determined.*

In an adult branch of a registration degree programme, time for reflection was built into the overall timetable. For example, at the start of the branch pro-gramme, students were given 1 week to reflect on the development of their learning:

Students who successfully complete the Common Foundation Programme will proceed to their selected branch programme and undertake an initial study week. During this time students will be provided with the opportunity to reflect upon knowledge and experience gained in the Common Foundation Programme in readiness for the transition to the Branch Programme.

The week will provide the student with the opportunity to reflect upon past experiences and individual progress and consider their own academic and professional development within the branch programme.

This approach could also be identified in post-registration courses. For exam-ple, in an ENB-approved post-registration course for advanced work with peo-ple with learning disabilities, an evaluative case study formed the major part of the assessment. This assessment was based on reflection on practice in the following way:

❖ *Using data from reflective diaries, introduces the client, and sets the scene, identifies the problems facing the client, and the mental health problems which present, and/or the behaviours which are currently challenging carers and/or service providers (10%)*

◆ *Documenting the process of assessment and functional analysis, rationalising decisions made and proposing an hypothesis. (Data collected should be included as appendices) (40%)*

◆ *A critical analysis of the interventions selected to address the client's needs, including a literature based rationale. The study should indicate the nursing framework/model that is to be used (50%).*

Reflection in practice

The importance which lecturers attached to the development of reflection meant that they saw student-centred teaching as a mechanism for drawing on and enhancing practical skills and personal experience which could contribute to a general understanding of risk issues. For example, a lecturer for the learning disability branch of a registration degree said that he approached risk teaching in the following way:

The best thing ... is to make it real by discussing case scenarios, preferably try and lift something out of their own experiences, e.g. if they were doing cooking classes with someone and something happened then they could think about it and analyse the risk components.

A lecturer on the adult branch of a registration degree who felt that students' 'own life experiences' were central to their perceptions and understanding of risk, used critical incidents as a way of enhancing students' understanding:

I think they (critical incidents) must be one of the best ways of learning because students can look at, they can analyse the incident, apply their theoretical knowledge but also they can go over the incident and think 'Did I behave?' 'Was the way I intervened appropriate?' 'Could I have done it another way?' – It's not judgmental in a negative way. It's a way of trying to help them become independent practitioners in the way that isn't making them feel that they've made mistakes all the time because we all make mistakes and there's so many situations that could go one way one day and one way the next. It's so unpredictable.

Another important teaching method was the use of diaries, to enable and encourage students to reflect on practice. In some courses, there were formal sessions in which students were invited to draw on incidents which they had recorded as a way of reflecting on practice. The same lecturer remarked that:

They record all kinds of things from their own vulnerability in situations, that they didn't know what to say, or what to do – sometimes it's practical things, sometimes it's the actual nature of nursing, sometimes it's power relationships.

All respondents saw reflection on practice as a major source of learning about risk. Although mentors tended to emphasise the importance of placements as the basis of learning from experience, they were also willing to recognise the importance of reflection on experience in college.

For lecturers, learning about risk was an integral part of the general process of learning to reflect on practice. Thus, they drew attention to the opportunities provided in college to reflect on experiences. A lecturer on a learning disability branch of a registration diploma course pointed to the following opportunities for student learning:

> *Role play – discussion, problem based learning. [Students are] given a scenario of a risk based dilemma [and] may also look at different ethical issues and look at nursing outcome and intervention.*

A lecturer on a mental health branch of a registration diploma course identified a similar range of learning opportunities:

> *Researcher:* How do you think students learn about risk then?
> *Lecturer:* I think predominantly by coming across it. I think it's also their greatest fears …. It's a theme that comes right from the beginning. They generate it in the examples they choose to use in critical incidents. They generate it when we're doing video work and interpersonal work, role play, it's nearly always about the fears of what might happen in their responsibilities …. I'd like to think we actually look at some of the research and some of the things, the current work that's been published on it.

Students recognised the opportunities provided by reflection on practice in class but saw it very much in the context of and as an extension of practice:

> *Researcher:* How do you think you learn about risk?
> *Student:* Doing it – learning by your mistakes. Learning from examples of other staff. Reflection. Critical incident analysis – it does help you reflect. If you're asked a question – on-going assignments – what would happen if this was happening. Being able to question your own actions.

All participants felt that practice was the main source of student learning about risk. Respondents identified different ways of learning. Some respondents valued learning which came from specific structuring of practice, such as opportunities to participate in or observe specific types of decisions; we refer to this as structured learning. Others respondents saw risk learning as integral to the general placement experience and as having a chance element; we refer to this as experiential learning.

Learning about risk from practice

Mentors argued that risk was best taught through structured practice. For example, a mentor for students on the mental health branch of a diploma registration programme commented on the limitations of class teaching and the importance of properly structured placements for effective learning:

> *Researcher:* How do you think students learn about risk?
>
> *Mentor:* Sometimes the hard way. It's something that's not easy to teach in a classroom setting .... In classrooms it always revolves around suicide because that's the big thing and around harm to others .... I do think that means that other risks aren't identified and I think that very often students learn about risk from their placements on the ward and I think it depends how those placements are constructed how quickly they learn about risk. Because if, as has been my experience in one area, they were having a day a week for so many weeks, they weren't learning anything because nobody took them seriously, their presence didn't count, they weren't there long enough to gel, they were a visitor every week. Whereas, I think if they have 3 or 4 days a week and they work as part of that team, they get the information they need. They learn about risk first-hand from various disciplines' perspectives. They become involved in discussions at ward rounds and at handovers ... they're able to reflect and attach risk to other situations they've either seen or been in.

The opportunities for learning depended on the ways in which placements were organised and supervised. The nature of structuring varied. In early stages of registration training, practice teachers saw themselves as playing an active role and ascribed a relatively passive observational role to students. A mentor for students on the adult branch of a registration degree described learning in the following way:

> *There's a certain trial and error. We prepare the students as best we can for going out there and we highlight, when they're at the junior level, the necessity for being an observer and a participant under observation, so that [if] they're taking actions [they are] guided by the mentor.*

Towards the end of registration courses and in post-registration courses, students were expected to play a more active role, with the mentor providing advice and guidance. In one mental health branch diploma course the placements were structured around a care group approach, so that students took responsibility for the care of a group of clients under the supervision of an appropriately qualified practice teacher. This was described in course documentation in the following way:

> *The student will build up a caseload of clients with a variety of mental health problems that reflects the demographic realities of mental health services provided for communities. This enables the student to be involved in the care of a number of clients over an extended period of time that would not otherwise be possible within the time constraints of more traditional approaches to clinical placements. The students' involvement with clients will be for variable periods of time reflecting the needs of both the client and the student. Over a period of time the constitution of the care group will change, due to turnover of the clients involved.*

Most respondents recognised that students' own activities and interpretation of their experiences were major factors in learning. Their contribution was described by one mentor in the following way:

> *By being in the job and seeing the situations for themselves. It's always been that way. You can talk about it and talk about it until you're blue in the face but, until you actually do it, the finer points of risks and risk taking won't actually sink in. They certainly didn't when I was doing my training, until you actually got on to the wards and you saw what they meant, you could use all the theoretical basis and the theoretical knowledge that you have but until you were out there doing the job you didn't actually understand most of what it meant.*

Students accepted this situation as they did not see risk as part of theory and therefore did not believe it was possible to learn about risk in class. For them risk assessment and management were primarily practical skills which they learned in practice and from personal experience. Indeed, they saw learning from practice and from experience as interconnected, and considered that practice formed part of their developing personal experience. Two students felt that they learned about risk in the following ways:

Researcher: How do you think you learn about risk?
Student A: From practice – seeing situations on placement.
Student B: Getting people out of bed you come across risk.

The students felt that practice was the main place where they learned about risk. Students on the adult branch of a registration degree made the following comments:

Researcher: How do you think you learn about risk?
Student A: ...you can't learn it until you have experienced it in a real life situation.

Student B: You're put into scenarios in the university but it's not until you've been in that scenario that you learn because you're drawing on the knowledge of other staff. You're thinking on your feet.

Student C: We've just had experience of running a team and have been well supported on the ward and in the university.

Student A: You can discuss management but until you're involved it doesn't happen.

Student C: On the ward there's always someone to fall back on.

Although students accepted that practice was an effective place for learning about risk, they felt that their opportunity to learn was affected by the ways in which their practice teachers defined their role and structured the placement. One district nursing student stated:

I've had a superb CPT (clinical placement teacher) and I've learnt more from her than I've ever learnt in my career.

However, some students felt that when their involvement was restricted to observation and they could not really learn:

Perhaps you learn from observations – from role models as you're going through. Seeing how other people manage things and you pick it up from there. It's certainly trial and error.

One group of students recognised that there was a variety of opportunities for learning but were concerned that there were no checks on whether these opportunities were used by individual students:

Student: [There is] no formal seminar entitled risk management but you just take it as a part of the course when on placement and discuss it with your mentor. But there are no guidelines for you to do it – nobody would know if you hadn't done it.

Researcher: What about in legal and ethics module?

Student: Possibly – when we've been given a scenario case when the nurse was accountable. But it's an optional module; you don't have to take it.

Some students suggested that risk teaching was like being taught to swim by being thrown in at the deep end of a swimming pool. They were expected to learn from their mistakes but were provided with limited support. For example, a mature student on an adult branch of a diploma registration course who had already completed a professional course made the following observation:

I see myself as fairly exceptional because I've already completed a professional training course so I can see the holes in the training. What the teachers think carries on is not always the case. A lot is implied. They expect you to pick up a lot of things and people who don't have my background may not be picking up on these cues ... the practicality is that you're thrown in at the deep end and you learn risk assessment on the job but there is still a massive gap between theory and practice.

Learning from personal experience

Most respondents felt that students did not just learn about risk from structured opportunities provided in practice but learnt from their general or personal experience. This could be in the clinical setting. For example, a group of students on the adult branch of a registration degree discussed risk learning in the following way:

Student A: Sometimes from mistakes if one takes little risks and those you see or hear about. Sometimes from others' mistakes. You learn by experience talking to ward staff – they can advise you and tell you about their experiences.

Student B: When you start out you don't realise you're taking risks – you're quite naïve.

While a student on an ENB post-registration course for the care of older people commented:

Trial and error when you're first qualified. You may handle a situation in one way and learn from that.

However, more often it was from general life experiences. Some teachers argued that, since risk was part of everyday life, individuals had to develop their own personal strategies for assessing and managing risk. One mental health lecturer described her personal strategy in the following way:

Being the woman in the street – my personal life and how it is influenced. I wouldn't walk round (the) City centre at three o'clock in the morning on my own. Risk is important and influences and affects life. Risk is an inexact concept – what might be my risk is not yours. It's about safety, suicide, violence, self-neglect, self-harm.

Some lecturers saw this form of teaching as a progression from and development of reflective practice. For example, one responded to the question about the risk teaching in the following way:

Discussion and reflective practice. There comes a point when you let them go and make their own mistakes. Not to put them in at the deep end – they are cossetted to a degree but you realise you have to let them go. In the past people have learnt quickly from demonstration but now we're producing nurses who are questioning practice. Patients must have been put at risk before when you think we just did things but didn't question.

Some students emphasised the continuity between learning on the course and learning in their personal life. A group of students on a post-registration ENB course for the care of older people commented on risk learning in the following way:

Researcher. How do you think you learn about risk?

Student A: Experience.

Student B: From being a baby you're taught about risk. If you put your finger near the fire it's moved away – so all along you're taught about risks – it's in-bred in you that you need to be cautious about certain things.

A similar approach was taken by students on the mental health branch of a registration degree:

Researcher. How do you think you learn about risk, you've had some teaching haven't you?

Student A: Just by being presented with situations which might cause you a dilemma over whether you're going to take a risk or not but that's not just in the work setting, it's in your own personal life I think how you learn about.

Student B: I mean you're up against risks all the time, making decisions is a risk.

COMMENT

Respondents identified a variety of opportunities for students to learn about risk: in college, in clinical placement and in their everyday life. There was agreement amongst respondents that students learnt from practice, either from observation or supervised practice or through the general process of decision making and the associated process of learning by trial and error.

There are some limitations with this approach to learning. There was a chance or random element in some of the learning. It was not clear whether all students had the same learning opportunities and whether all students had the ability to exploit the opportunities provided. Furthermore, given the lack of formal and explicit assessment of students' competence in risk assessment and management, it was not clear how lecturers and mentors ensured all students had the requisite competences.

Through their education nurses should acquire the appropriate knowledge, skills and attitudes to competently provide care and to effectively assess and manage risk. The nurses in our study saw knowledge as the key to effective risk management and decision making so the key element of educational preparation was the acquisition of appropriate knowledge. It is clear that nurses also saw risk management and decision making in terms of technical skills, but since the skills were not explicitly identified, nurses were expected to acquire them in practice. It is possible that Benner's view (1984) that experienced nurses internalise such skills and use intuition justifies this approach but, as we have argued in this book, there are complex technical elements of risk management and decision making that can and should be explicitly taught. It is not clear from our study that most nurses saw risk management in terms of values. Nurses are evidently provided with education that draws attention to values but the link between values and risk does not appear to be clearly established. It is to these issues we now turn in the concluding chapter.

Risk, trust and nursing: towards an ethical basis for risk assessment and management in practice

Andy Alaszewski

INTRODUCTION

In this chapter we summarise and develop our overall analysis of the ways in which nurses manage risk and identify ways in which nursing practice can be developed. We start by reconsidering the problems posed by risk assessment, communication and management in nursing practice; we then explore the issue of risk in decision making and its implications for informed consent; and, finally, we examine the ethical basis of risk assessment and management in nursing practice.

THE ROLE OF PROFESSIONALS: CREATING

SECURITY AND SUSTAINING TRUST

Health and welfare agencies and their professional employees have a crucial role to play in modern society. They have the responsibility for providing individuals with both individual and collective security and protection. Thus, professionals seek to identify the causes of harm and counteract them. As Green pointed out in her historical analysis of 'accidents', epidemiologists have sought to convert unpredictable and therefore uncontrollable 'accidents' into predictable and therefore potentially controllable 'risks':

> *By the end of the twentieth century, the accidental itself had become a central focus, as the ultimate challenge for risk technologies. To predict the unpredictable, and make random misfortune preventable was a notable success of epidemiology.* (Green, 1999: 37).

However, both professionals and the users of their services recognise that it is impossible to prevent all harm. Death may be seen as the ultimate harm; however, it is inevitable that all individuals will eventually die. So, if and when death becomes inevitable, the focus of professional interest should shift to meeting the needs of the dying person such as enabling the individual to die with as much dignity as possible.

The issue is not death or harm but premature death or preventable harm. Thus, we have argued that professionals should not aim to prevent all harm but rather they should seek to minimise it. Such an approach is both realistic and essentially empowering, as it respects the service user's values:

> *Although harm reduction strategies are being promoted essentially for pragmatic reasons and as the 'least bad alternative' (Strang and Farrell, 1992), it is also possible to identify a rational, even utopian element within them. They aim to create a better and a safer society by directly and immediately reducing harm and indirectly, in the longer term, reducing the overall incidence of harmful behaviours. They are rational in so far as they are concerned with identifying causes and basing interventions on analysis of the reasons for actions. However unlike more idealistic approaches, they do not attempt to re-engineer the individual by taking away his or her choice to engage in behaviours such as alcohol consumption or illicit drug use, rather they are more concerned with identifying and changing the specific aspects of these behaviours that cause harm.* (Alaszewski et al., 1998b: 143).

Harm minimisation strategies can be seen as a partnership between service users and professionals based on trust. Professionals need to respect the service user's value system and right to make decisions based on these values if others are not harmed even if they result in activities which the professional does not agree with, such as using illicit drugs or 'natural childbirth'. Users have to be confident that the information which professionals provide, especially about the nature of hazards and potential harm, is objective, based on evidence and does not contain implicit values and judgements.

Thus, harm minimisation strategies need to be based on a trusting relationship in which risks are shared. The expert provides information on the probable consequences of different courses of actions and the service user can then make an informed choice. The risk for professionals is that the service user will chose a course of action which in their opinion is not likely to result in the best outcome. The risk for users is that their desired and intended outcome will not be achieved. However, this approach does have advantages: for the user it involves empowerment, although it is important to note that not all users will want or be able to take responsibility; for the professional, it involves sharing responsibility and, if something goes wrong and serious harm occurs, avoiding the blame.

When things go wrong and serious harm results, professionals tend to be blamed if it can be shown that they influenced the decision by providing biased information or by withholding important information. In the case of paediatric open heart surgery in Bristol, parents providing consent for the operation were not informed that over half the children did not survive the operation. The consequences of betrayal of trust which occur when information and risk are not shared can be devastating not only for service users but also for the professionals and the agencies which employ them. In the Bristol case the paediatric heart surgeon involved, Mr Wisheart, and the chief executive of the hospital trust, Dr John Roylance, were both struck off the medical register while the trust has made payments of £50,000 to the parent(s) of each child who died and will have to make substantial payments to provide for the care of the brain damaged and disabled children.

The government's response to the Bristol disaster and other similar cases has been to make the chief executives of NHS trusts accountable to Parliament for the quality of clinical decisions from 1 April 1999 through clinical governance (Millar, 1999: 22). However, the precise nature and meaning of clinical governance is elusive. The departmental document which announced clinical governance not only failed to define it but also placed it alongside professional self-regulation without specifying how and in what ways the two processes were linked:

> *The Government will help to ensure national quality standards are applied consistently within local practice through a new system of clinical governance: through extended life-long learning to ensure that NHS staff are equipped to deliver change and are given opportunity to maintain their skills and expertise, and through modernised professional self-regulation.*
>
> *Clinical governance will be the process by which each part of the NHS quality-assures its clinical decisions. Backed by a new statutory duty of quality, clinical governance will introduce a system of continuous improvements into the NHS ....*

Professional self-regulation provides clinicians with the opportunity to help set standards. People need to be confident that the regulatory bodies will exercise rigorous self-regulation over the standard and conduct of health professionals and will act promptly and openly when things go wrong. The Government is committed to working with the professional regulatory bodies to ensure that professional self-regulation keeps pace with public expectations and is more open and accountable. For example, a modernised regulatory system will play a fuller part in the early identification of possible lapses in clinical quality. (NHS Executive, 1999: 2–3).

Central government appears to want to reassure the public by placing a legal responsibility on chief executives for the quality of clinical decisions and at the same time to reassure the medical profession that it would be retaining its autonomy. A cynic might argue that the government wanted to have its cake and to eat it too. The apparent tension between clinical governance and professional self-regulation can only be resolved if there is collaboration between managers and professionals and it is therefore not surprising to find the main architects of the proposals arguing that:

The strength of the working relationship between senior managers and health professionals will be at the heart of clinical governance. (Scally and Donaldson, 1998: 63).

If this occurs then it is possible that the government may succeed in reversing the trend and increase the public trust in the NHS and the professional staff it employs by providing two separate but mutually reinforcing mechanisms of assurance. The use of the term 'trust' as the name for the organisations providing care and treatment indicates the importance placed on this ideal.

The absence of central guidance on clinical governance has created a vacuum that has been partially filled by the NHS itself, through workshops and commentaries. The central concept of clinical governance continues to be slippery but it is clear that there are links to risk assessment and management. For example, North Thames Region organised eight workshops and these drew attention to the danger of developing a defensive, risk-averse 'blame and shame' culture (NHS Executive, 1999: 1). Barbara Millar's (1999) survey of senior managers in the NHS identified the importance of 'clear procedures aimed at managing risk' (Millar 1999: 23). Several participants in her study made an explicit link between clinical governance and risk issues. The Chief Executive of Mid Sussex Trust commented that:

Initially, there will be a lot more defensive clinical practice .... I think practitioners will be far less prepared to work at the perceived margins of safety ... [Prevent another Bristol]. It may be less likely. But human nature and the sheer size of the health service mean that we will never have a defect and error-free NHS. (Millar, 1999: 27).

The chief nurse at University College London Hospitals clearly identified the role of clinical governance in providing reassurance:

[Prevent another Bristol] No. I wish I could say it would, but it's Sod's law that if it can happen, it will. But it [clinical governance] will reassure politicians and the public that there are more overt mechanisms in place than ever before. (Millar, 1999: 26).

It is clear that trust is central to the management of health care in general and risk in particular, and that the interactions between professionals and their clients are influenced by and impact on the development of trust. Since trust may be easy to destroy and difficult to build, we turn in the next section to the ways in which trust can be developed.

DEVELOPING AND ENHANCING TRUST: COMMUNICATION AND RESPECT

In this book we have been concerned with the ways in which nurses and other professionals can build and sustain trust. It is clear that trust can be developed and enhanced if there is a partnership between nurses, the agencies which employ them and the clients or patients who use their services. These relationships exist for a purpose; in the case of the health service, this purpose is the treatment of patients. Underpinning these relationships are decisions about treatment, and if patients are to have trust in the nurses who care for them and the agencies which provide the care, then they must have confidence in the quality of the decision-making process.

As we pointed out in Chapters 4 and 5, very little attention has been paid to the nature of nurses' decision making. It seems self-evident that a starting point for the evaluation of professional decision making in general and nurses' decision making in specific should be the impact of decisions on services. 'Good' decisions are those which effectively manage risk by maximising benefit and minimising harm to service users and others (Vincent, 1997). It is relatively easy to assess serious harm such as death and it seems self-evident that better decisions result in lower levels of harm. This approach builds on well-established approaches to evaluating clinical practice and fits well with other initiatives being taken by the current government, such as National Standards and guidelines of new evidence-based National Service Frameworks and the National Institute for Clinical Excellence. Indeed, one of the obvious indicators of the scale of the disaster at Bristol was the level of harm to patients. An independent review of 53 operations undertaken by the paediatric heart surgeon identified an unacceptably high level of harm, 29 deaths (see Boseley, 1999a: 6).

Such approaches will build on earlier systems of prevention and harm minimisation such as those lying in professional self-regulation, the UKCC's code and associated guidelines of professional conduct and practice. The guidelines for professional practice clearly identify nurses' duty to protect the users of their services. This is referred to as the 'duty of care' and is specified in the following way:

> *You [the registered nurse] have both a legal and a professional duty to care for patients and clients. In law, the courts could find a registered practitioner negligent if a person suffers harm because he or she failed to care for them properly. Professionally, the UKCC's Professional Conduct Committee could find a registered practitioner guilty of misconduct and remove them from the register if he or she failed to care properly for a patient or client, even though they suffered no harm .... If there is a complaint against you, the UKCC's Professional Conduct Committee and possibly the courts would decide whether you took proper care. When they do this, they must consider whether what you did was reasonable in all the circumstances.* (UKCC, 1996: 10).

The importance of harm minimisation is reinforced by the first two clauses of the Code of Professional Conduct:

> *As a registered nurse, midwife or health visitor, you are personally accountable for your practice and, in the exercise of your professional accountability, must:*
>
> 1 *act always in such a manner as to promote and safeguard the interests and well-being of patients and clients;*
> 2 *ensure that no action or omission on your part, or within your sphere of responsibility, is detrimental to the interests, condition or safety of patients and clients ....* (UKCC, 1992).

However, focussing on the outcome and using it to identify and differentiate 'good' from 'bad' decisions may be unhelpful. As Dowie (1999) argued, in practice it is more helpful to focus on the decision-making process and therefore on 'better' and 'worse' decisions. In the case of the Bristol disaster, media attention was related to the scale of the disaster, the level of preventable harm and the status of the 'victims' – highly vulnerable babies and their parents. The actual inquiry has concentrated on the underlying cause of this harm – the defects in the decision-making process. This is in line with the parents' complaints, which were about the decision-making process and, in particular, that they were deprived of the opportunity of making informed consent. They were aware that the operations were risky but not quite how risky. As one parent put it:

> *Had we known of the real statistics we would never have accepted the referral .... When I signed the consent form I believed I was doing the best thing for Mia. However, in retrospect I know that I did not. I maintain that my consent to this operation was obtained by giving me false information. This is in my view criminal.* (Quoted in Boseley, 1999b).

Users and carers want full information, so that they can fully participate in the decision-making process. As Myers and MacDonald noted in their discussion of the involvement of older users and their carers in decision making: if professionals only provide limited information, then users and carers are presented with options rather than given full choice (Myers and MacDonald, 1996: 104–9).

The importance of involving service users in the process of decision making is well recognised and is acknowledged within the professional Code of Conduct. For example, the UKCC provides separate guidelines for nurses working with people with mental illness and with learning disabilities. This guidance stresses the importance of user participation in the following way:

> *The registered practitioner must not practise in a way which assumes that only they know what is best for the patient or client, as this can only create a dependence and interfere with the patient's or client's right to choose.*
>
> *Advocacy is concerned with promoting and protecting the interests of patients or clients, many of whom may be vulnerable and incapable of protecting their own interests and who may be without the support of family or friends. You can do this by providing information and making the patient or client feel confident that he or she can make their own decisions.*
>
> *Advocacy also involves providing support if the patient refuses treatment/care or withdraws their consent. Other health care professionals, families, legal advisers, voluntary agencies and advocates appointed by the courts may also be involved in safeguarding the interests of patients and clients.*
>
> *Respect for patients' and clients' autonomy means that you should respect the choices they make concerning their own lives. Clause 5 of the code outlines your professional role in promoting patient/client independence. This means discussing with them any proposed treatment or care so that they can decide whether to refuse or accept that treatment or care. This information should enable the patient or client to decide what is in their own best interests.* (UKCC, 1996: 13–14).

This guidance also recognises the problems created by mental incapacity and that nurses need to use their judgement in such circumstances:

Registered practitioners must respect patients' and clients' rights to take part in decisions about their care. You must use your professional judgement, often in conjunction with colleagues, to decide when a patient or client is capable of making an informal decision about his or her treatment and care. If possible, the patient or client should be able to make a choice about his or her care, even if this means that they may refuse care. You must make sure that all decisions are based on relevant knowledge. The patients' or clients' right to agree to or to refuse treatment and care may change in law depending on their age and health (refer to the section on consent). Particular attention to the legal position of children must be given, as their right to give consent or refuse treatment or care varies in different parts of the United Kingdom and depending on their age. (UKCC, 1996: 14).

The UKCC sees risk management as one response to the tensions involved:

The risk management process should enable the optimum level of care to be given to a client. Risk management involves the assessment of risk relating to client care, care systems and the environment of care. The calculation of risk must be based on your knowledge, skills and competence and you are accountable for your actions and omissions. You should value the process of risk taking, following assessment and in the context of appropriate management, as it will increase your ability to help clients to achieve their potential. However, you should be aware that there may be conflicts between your professional accountability and the autonomy of the client. Although it is rarely possible to eliminate risk entirely, you are still responsible for attempting to reduce risk to an agreed acceptable level. This level should be agreed within the inter-disciplinary team and, where possible, with the client. (UKCC, 1998: 22).

The UKCC does not provide guidance on how conflicts between professional accountability for safety and the autonomy should be resolved nor does it indicate how agreement over 'acceptable levels' of risk are to be established. It is clear that nurses have to exercise professional judgement, but the precise basis of this judgement is not clear and it is to this issue we turn in the final section of this chapter.

DEVELOPING AN ETHICAL BASIS FOR RISK MANAGEMENT AND DECISION MAKING

Information is clearly important in decision making and risk management but as we pointed out in Chapter 4 not all issues can be resolved by more or better information. The exercise of professional judgement, especially in the context of conflicts of interest and/or values, should be grounded in ethical principles, what is right or wrong, rather than pragmatism, what works or doesn't work. It is therefore important that nurses are aware of the ethical basis of their decision making and risk management and in this section we will consider three alternative ethical frameworks: utilitarianism, the human rights approach and the virtues approach.

As Plant (1991: 139) pointed out, the development of utilitarianism was a response to social change at the end of the 18th century, and in particular the decline of traditional communities with strong kin and personal ties, accepted custom and practice and shared religion all of which contributed to a taken-for-granted moral universe. What was right and wrong was easily and clearly defined. The development of modern society disrupted both traditional communities and their moral underpinning (for a classic analysis see Durkheim, 1952). The large-scale movements of populations associated with the development of money-based capitalist economies created large population concentrations in cities. As Plant noted:

> *people were uprooted from settled moral communities and thrust into new relationships with strangers .... Individuals [in modern society] confront one another without clear expectations, they can no longer rely on the moral assumptions and habits of a lifetime ....* (Plant, 1991: 139).

Utilitarianism was an attempt to fill the vacuum created by the destruction of the shared moral values of traditional communities. It started from a recognition that individuals in modern society had different value systems and should be able to use these to define their own wants and preferences: in Bentham's terms, their own happiness. The focus of utilitarianism is on the values which should underpin collective decisions, such as which individuals should receive services funded from taxes. Bentham argued that the only ethical basis for collective action was the 'greatest happiness of the greatest number' (Bentham, 1982: 13; see also 282) or the maximisation of the overall welfare of the population. The individual should be the judge of his or her own happiness; thus, utilitarianism both recognises and respects individual value systems. Rawls provided the following summary of utilitarianism:

> *The main idea is that society is rightly ordered, and therefore just, when its major institutions are arranged so as to achieve the greatest net balance of satisfaction summed over all the individuals belonging to it.* (Rawls, 1972: 22).

Two immediate difficulties can be identified with this approach. The first is technical – how to assess, measure and aggregate 'satisfaction' or happiness of different individuals. The second is perhaps more fundamental. If a specific community is divided into two unequal-sized groups with differentiated and incompatible value systems, then applying the 'greatest happiness of the greatest number' formula may result in the repression of the minority by the majority. For example, as MacIntyre pointed out, it is difficult to see the application of the principle in which 'public happiness is found by the public itself to consist of the mass murder of Jews' (MacIntyre, 1967: 238). Another way of making the same point is to consider the situation of two nonsmokers who have to share an office with 10 individuals who smoke. In England, utilitarianism has been used to justify the repression of minorities. For example, Bentham himself was actively concerned with the design of prisons (Semple, 1993), while one of his followers, Chadwick, was a major architect of the 1834 Poor Law Amendment Act, a repressive response to the threat of the rural poor (Checkland and Checkland, 1974). As Rawls pointed out, utilitarianism can easily slip into bureaucratic efficiency, with good decisions being equated with the efficient management of social problems (Rawls, 1972: 27).

It is possible to identify a utilitarian element in current approaches to health, especially in public health. The technical problems of measurement apply particularly to positive aspects of welfare. It is difficult to measure pleasure or happiness. However, Bentham also recognised negative elements: in his terms, pain, or in risk terms, harm. Harm to individuals is easier to define, measure and compare, for in health there are well-established measures of mortality and morbidity. These appear to provide a clear moral basis for decisions which command wide support. Harm is self-evidently bad and the goal of public action should be to minimise harm, illness and death. The utilitarian underpinning of current health policy can be clearly seen in the Labour government's policy statement on public health entitled *Saving Lives,* where the goals of public health were specified in the following way:

◆ to improve the health of the population as a whole by increasing the length of people's lives and the number of years people spend free from illness; and
◆ to improve the health of the worst off in society and to narrow the gap. (Department of Health, 1999: para 1.17).

The White Paper identified the potential for harm minimisation through a reduction in mortality:

> *by cutting needless early deaths from cancer, coronary heart disease and stroke, accidents and suicide, there is the real prospect of reducing the number of deaths from these causes by up to 300,000 by the year 2010.* (Department of Health, 1999: para 1.17).

Thus, the overall aims of public health policy identified in an earlier policy document *Our Healthier Nation* are the minimisation of harm where possible, and its fair distribution when it cannot be avoided:

A healthy country would be one where health was not dictated by accident of birth and childhood experience. Everyone should have a fair chance of long and healthy life …. The poorest in our society are hit harder than the well off by most of the major causes of death. (Department of Health, 1998a: 9).

Utilitarianism can be helpful in decisions which affect large groups of individuals and, in particular, decisions which affect the allocation of resources between individuals or between groups. At practice level some of the decisions which community nurses and community teams make can be seen as resource allocation or rationing decisions: for example, when teams decide to accept one eligible referral but not another or individual nurses decide to visit one client and not another who could benefit from their services, they are making implicit rationing decisions. In this context it is clearly important to consider the utility or benefit generated by different courses of action. Although such decisions are important, the ones that most concern individual nurses are those which relate to individual users, and here utilitarianism does not provide any guidance. Utilitarianism is based on the assumption that individuals can define and pursue their own wants. Indeed it:

conflates all persons into one through the imaginative acts of the impartial sympathetic spectator. Utilitarianism does not take seriously the distinction between persons. (Rawls, 1972: 27).

It is precisely this distinction between people that nurses are interested in when they make decisions. They are concerned with the unique characteristics of each individual and situation and they need to be able to assess their decisions in terms of their impact on specific unique individuals. Thus, they need some ethical basis for judging the impact of their actions on the individuals who use their services.

One approach to this individual level is through the concept of human or natural rights in which all individuals are seen as possessing certain basic rights and that:

men are entitled to make certain claims by virtue simply of their common humanity. (MacDonald, 1984: 21).

This approach has a long tradition and can be traced back to the Greeks and the Romans but 'tends to be renewed at every crisis in human affairs' (MacDonald, 1984: 21). The political and social crises at the end of the 18th century in Europe and North America provided a major stimulus. Like utilitarianism, the human rights approach was an attempt to identify a moral basis for society to replace traditional systems. While utilitarians such as Chadwick sought to transform society through radical administrative reform, human rights activists advocated revolutionary action designed to destroy tradition-al 'despotic' political systems and replace them with modern, purpose-designed 'democratic' systems. For example, Paine devoted the first part of his treatise on the *Rights of Man*, first published in 1792, to defending the French Revolution and the second part to the lessons that could be learnt from the new Republic of the United States of America created by the 'American Revolution'. For Paine the key feature and strength of these new systems was that they had formal and agreed statements, constitutions, which clearly and explicitly defined the civil rights of all members of society and identified mechanisms to protect such rights. Indeed, protecting such rights was the basis and justification of the system:

> *Civil rights are those which appertain to man [sic] in right of his being a member of society. Every civil right has for its foundation some natural right pre-existing in the individual, but to the enjoyment of which his individual power is not, in all cases, sufficiently competent. Of this kind are all those which relate to security and protection.* (Paine, 1921: 44).

Both the French Republic and the United States of America made declarations based on individual civil liberties:

> *'Men are born free and equal,' said the French Assembly, 'in respect of their* natural *and* imprescriptible *rights of liberty, property, security, and resistance to oppression.' The framers of the American Declaration of Independence declare as self-evident truths that all men are created equal, that they are endowed by their creator with inalienable rights, among which are Life, Liberty, and the Pursuit of Happiness, and that governments are instituted to secure these rights.* (Normal type shows emphasis in the original, MacDonald, 1984: 27).

From these revolutionary origins, the concept of human and civil rights has become incorporated into the political mainstream and there have been moves to provide globalised or universal human rights:

> *The most recent political examples [of attempts to codify fundamental human rights include] the Universal Declaration of Human Rights adopted by the United Nations, which in its preamble is supposed to set 'a common standard of achievement for all peoples and all nations'.* (Plant, 1991: 255).

As Waldron pointed out, given the wide variety of 'inhumane' practices that are accepted in different parts of the world (Waldron, 1984: 3), the key ques-tion is how are universal rights defined. Various commentators have tried to list natural rights. For example, Maritain has listed rights to life, liberty, property, and to pursue a religious vocation, marry and raise a family and to be treated as a person and not as a thing (cited in MacDonald, 1984: 31).

The 19th century philosopher John Stuart Mill argued that rights were basic interests which needed to be protected to ensure individual existence:

> *These basic interests are, in Mill's view, of two sorts: physical nutriment and general security of person and possession. These are the necessary goods, or interests of all human beings ... we have a claim on our fellow citizens to 'join in making safe the very groundwork of our existence'.* (Plant, 1991: 165).

Given the influence of the concept of human rights, it is hardly surprising that they should be seen as a framework for decision making in health care. In the early 1990s, the British government published its Patient's Charter. This Charter was presented as an agreed structure for NHS/citizen relations, specifying the rights of individuals to services and the standards which they could expect. The 1995 version of the Charter grouped overall rights and standards into three main sections: access to services; personal consideration and respect; and the provision of information (Department of Health, 1995: 5–7). It is therefore possible to identify three basic principles: the provision of security for individuals, through appropriate access to services and treatment; recognition of and respect for individual diversity, including individual value systems; and the provision of information, so that individuals can make informed choices. Given the importance of the rights approach it is hardly surprising that these three principles are also the ones which we identified as underpinning nursing ethics. The problem we identified in the last section of how to make a decision when there is conflict between different rights is not resolved.

One possible approach to this problem is for nurses to adopt a counselling approach to decision making and grant primacy to the user's right to information. In the counselling mode, the responsibility of the nurse is to provide the service user with information about risk, about the probability of different consequences. The user is treated as a rational person who uses this information to make choices. In the counselling approach, counsellors have to accept that users may not share their values and, in particular, may not define harm and security in a similar way or give them the same priority.

This approach is especially well developed in the area of genetic counselling (see Cunningham-Burley and Kerr, 1999). The rapid development of knowledge about human genetics has increased the accuracy of the assessment of the risks that a couple will have a child with a genetic disorder. This has stimulated the development of genetic counselling:

> *As knowledge about human genetic make-up accumulates, there is mounting pressure to expand existing genetic counselling services and increase the number of settings where genetic counselling is practiced.* (Petersen, 1999).

In view of the past abuses of genetics, especially those associated with the eugenic movements, the avowed aim of genetic counselling is to provide objective information so that individuals can make their own choices:

> Genetic counselling, it is argued, should be 'client-centred' and 'non-directive'. Counsellors should impart genetic risk information but withhold direct advice, enabling patients/clients to reach 'informed', voluntary decisions. (Petersen, 1999).

As advocates of the genetic counselling have argued, the primary aim of genetic counselling is not harm minimisation, preventing genetic disorder, although this may be a positivé by-product of the process:

> Genetic counselling does not aim to prevent couples from having children with genetic diseases. Preventing genetic disorders, although important, is secondary to good clinical practice, which identifies couples at risk and by empathic counselling allows them to make their own informed choice about prenatal diagnosis, termination of pregnancy or other aspects of management. Informed choice without external coercion should distinguish medical genetics from eugenics, which has the contrary aim of improving the communal gene pool. (Harris cited in Petersen, 1999).

Despite the explicit commitment to non-directive counselling, the reality is different. Hallowell, in a study of counselling about the hereditary risk of breast and ovarian cancer, showed that women using such services do not have autonomous choice. The women's choices were structured by the type of information they received:

> Given that individuals consider it important to present an image of behaving responsibly with regard to their health in general ... or genetic risk in particular ... the clinicians' portrayal of certain types of medical management as positive and responsible behaviour, may be interpreted as implicitly coercive. Opting for no further medical intervention is quite simply not an option, even for those at low risk ... in many sessions the clinicians failed to present the women with alternative courses of action ... even in those sessions in which the different risk management options were discussed, the clinicians' negative framing of particular options (ovarian screening, prophylactic mastectomy and no intervention) meant that they were not presented as viable or real alternatives. (Hallowell, 1999).

Lippman, using a 'rights' framework, argued that these limitations are so serious that choice and the counselling process, rather than empowering women, can become a threat to their welfare:

> Choice remains a fundamental necessity: it is both a basic civil right and a fundamental social right for all women .... Can I say no when asked if I

*want prenatal diagnosis without being made to feel culpable if I refuse
testing and a baby with Down syndrome is born .... If I have a problem
someone said I had the choice to avoid, I can then be held responsible for
having it ... agency without genuine autonomy is empty, and hazardous.*
(Lippman, 1999).

A fundamental problem in the rights approach in general and the counselling
approach specifically is the requirement to identify a 'person'. A person is a
'bearer' of rights who in counselling is responsible for judging his or her own
interests and making choices. Many ethical questions concern precisely this
issue. For example, should an unborn foetus have rights or what rights should
a person with dementia have? As Warnock pointed out, there is no objective
or universal definition of a person and each society has its own definition:

*Everyone who tries to come up with factual or scientific criteria for
personhood gets into difficulties over what we are to say about infants or
those who, though they once satisfied the criteria, are no longer able to do
so, such as those in a coma, or suffering from dementia. But this is not just
a little local difficulty. It is fundamental. For it is essentially for society to*
decide *who is a bearer of rights. There is no way of looking at the facts
about, say, a demented woman, and deducing whether she is a person.*
(Normal type shows emphasis in the original, Warnock, 1998: 55).

Both utilitarianism and the human rights approach can be used to inform
decision making and risk management, but both have limitations: utilitarianism is mainly concerned about group decisions, whereas rights are associated
with persons and cannot be used to define who and who is not a person. One
way out of this problem is to use the virtue approach originally developed by
Aristotle, the Greek philosopher. Aristotle argued that ethics is concerned
with 'good' and that good can be defined in relationship to the purpose or end
state of an action or thing:

*'Every craft and every inquiry, and similarly every action and project,
seems to aim at some good; hence the good has been well defined as that
at which everything aims' .... Good is defined at the outset in terms of the
goal, purpose, or aim to which something or somebody moves.* (MacIntyre,
1967: 57).

Thus, goodness is judged in terms of virtue, the quality of objects or activities
which contributed to an end state. For example, we can judge the quality of
a brick in terms of its contribution to a completed house or that of a musician
in terms of how his or her musical skills contribute to an overall musical
performance (Plant, 1991: 27–30). The object or person that achieves their
purpose can be seen as flourishing:

The notion of flourishing ... derives from the idea that every kind of object has its own essential end or function ... a musical instrument is for making music. The Greek word for excellence, arete is the word we translate as 'virtue'. So the excellence of a chair, a knife, a musical instrument, consists in its being able to fulfil its essential function (ergon) well. We might speak of an ideal chair, or an ideal knife, with approval. The idea that this generates, then, is that for an object or a creature to flourish, is for it to be in a state or situation that allows it to fulfil its essential function well. As far as human beings are concerned, this may well be a matter of displaying the traditional virtues. More broadly, however, flourishing may be taken as a matter of well-being or health in general, and the flourishing of animals and plants is easily graspable by analogy; the plant which has been left in a dark cellar, for example, metaphorically struggles to find the light it needs to blossom in its appropriate shape and colour – to become what we, as onlookers, know it can be, given the right conditions. (Almond, 2000).

The 'virtue' approach can be used to provide an ethical framework for making decisions about and managing the risk to individual health and welfare. Indeed, in one area in which risk management has been given particular prominence, the virtue approach is well developed. In child protection, social workers and other professionals have a legal duty to assess a child's risk of harm and to intervene when they judge this risk is significant or likely to become significant (see Lyon and de Cruz, 1993). The major criterion of harm is whether it prevents a child flourishing. This can be seen explicitly in relationship to babies with the identification of a 'failure to thrive' syndrome which can be defined in the following way:

Babies have an expected normal level of growth (weight and length), which is based upon their birth weight and size. Those that fall well below this expectation, with no apparent physical explanation, are considered to be causes for concern, and neglect (both physical and emotional) is thought to be a likely cause of this. Close monitoring of a child's physical growth when placed away from its parents may often show, that with reasonable care and feeding, normal development will take place, this proving that some form of neglect lies at the heart of the problem. (Corby, 1993: 46–7).

Although 'failure to thrive' is related specifically to babies, the broad approach is also adopted for all children. For example, in England, the Department of Health defined neglect in terms of:

significant impairment of the child's health or development, including non-organic failure to thrive. (Cited in Lyon and de Cruz, 1993: 6).

In Scotland, one local authority has provided a catalogue of the 'virtues' which an emotionally abused child may be deprived of:

> *Emotional abuse – This may result in over-anxiety in the child; avoidance of contacts outside the home; low self-esteem; limited capacity for enjoyment; serious aggression; impulsive behaviour; retardation of physical development through deprivation.* (Cited in Lyon and de Cruz, 1993: 6).

Failure to flourish underpins all areas of child protection. For example, the Children Act 1989 defines harm in terms of a child's:

> *'ill-treatment' or impairment of health and development.* (Cited in Freeman, 1994: 21).

Given the distinctive characteristics of child protection, with its emphasis on preventing harm and therefore its use of 'non-flourishing' as a measure of harm, it is not clear that this approach could and should be extended to other vulnerable groups living in the community. The use of the virtue approach would help fill a vacuum that is difficult to fill in any other way. For example, consider the following statement made by Nirje to support the claim that individuals with learning disabilities should have the right to self-determination:

> *If this right [to self determination] is not acknowledged and respected, if the retarded are not treated and met on that level, then the procedures described might become harmful and dangerous. If the problems and aspirations presented by the retarded adults are not dealt with realistically and with respect, but manipulated and essentially disregarded, then the persons treated this way will become injured and will experience the rejection and devaluation they have so often confronted.* (Nirje, 1972: 189).

Although Nirje used the rhetoric of rights, his statement can be interpreted within a 'virtue' framework. He claimed that a potential virtue of all individuals with learning disability is the ability to make decisions about their own future, and if they do not have this virtue then they do not flourish. Nirje justified this virtue in terms of contribution to a 'good' end state, for the individual the status of a person or citizen, and for society complete democracy:

> *when mentally retarded adults express their right to self-determination in public and in action, and thus gain and experience due citizen respect, they also have something to teach ... society in general; something about the deeper importance of democratic opportunities, the respect due to everyone in a democratic society – and that otherwise, democracy is not complete.* (Nirje, 1972: 189).

Focussing on virtues rather than rights has advantages. It avoids the question of whether an individual has or should have the status of a person; that is, someone capable of exercising rights. It avoids the 'all or nothing' approach of rights. If self-determination is treated as a right then an individual either does or does not have it. If it is treated as a virtue, then an individual can have more or less of it and action can be taken to increase or reduce it. Rights are treated as ends in themselves; for example, it is self-evidently good to have the right of self-determination. Virtues are essentially a means to an end and judged in terms of their contribution to that end: therefore, it is important in the virtues to define the ideal end – the state in which an individual flourishes.

It could be argued that defining the end or 'flourishing' state is difficult in respect of highly vulnerable or profoundly disabled people and their own views are rarely sought or responded to. However, in reality, judgements are made about desirable states. For example, in a classic study of the impact of deinstitutionalisation of children with learning disabilities, Tizard noted how they flourished as a result of their move into a family unit (Brooklands). The children:

> became able to play socially and constructively at a level approaching that
> of their mental age. Emotionally they became much less maladjusted … they
> developed strong attachments to members of staff and to other children.
> They were able to play co-operatively with other children, to take turns with
> as much grace as comparable normal children and to share. They were thus
> affectionate and happy children, usually busy and interested in what they
> were doing, confident and full of fun. In all these respects the behaviour of
> the children at Brooklands was in striking contrast to their earlier
> behaviour in the parent hospital, and to the behaviour of their peers who
> remained in the hospital. (Tizard, 1964: 133–4).

In this book there is also evidence that both carers and nurses on occasion used a virtue approach. In Chapter 3 we discussed the trust relationship between relatives of adults with learning disabilities and the staff of residential homes who took over prime responsibility for providing care. We argued that these families used the physical and mental well-being of their relative to judge the home. If their relative was frightened or had been physically injured, then they judged the care as inadequate; whereas if their relative appeared happy and in good health, they judged the care to be satisfactory. The relatives were making intuitive judgements about the virtues that they felt indicated a flourishing condition. We would argue that, currently, professionals are also intuitively making the same sort of judgements. We noted in Chapter 5 that nurses supporting vulnerable adults in the community devoted a considerable amount of time to visiting users in their own homes. During these visits, nurses assessed the users' conditions and in some circumstances decided that further action was necessary. We believe that these judgements are usually based on an assessment that the user is not flourishing, either on physical evidence of harm or on evidence of distress such as statements or actions that indicate fear or anxiety. Although some of these judgements are explicit and supported by evidence, such as the assessment of pressure sores of older service users, many are currently intuitive.

FINAL COMMENT

A prime responsibility of all nurses, but particularly nurses providing support for vulnerable individuals in the community, is to assess and manage risk. If they demonstrate that they are doing this effectively and systematically, they will gain and maintain the trust not only of individuals using their services but also of wider society.

There is a technical component to risk assessment and management. Nurses need to be able to show that they have relevant knowledge, or in current parlance, the relevant evidence, and need to be able to demonstrate that they can use this knowledge appropriately.

However, there is more to decision making and risk management than technical efficiency. Given the broader social context of risk management and decision making – for example, harm created by the failure to effectively assess and manage risk may fall on innocent victims – it is important that nurses are able to convince others that their decisions are fair and just. To do this they need to be able to demonstrate that their decision making and risk management have an ethical basis.

Currently, most risk management is viewed in an essentially pragmatic way, using an implicit utilitarian approach of minimising individual and collective harm. We have argued that nurses can and should develop a more sophisticated approach and that the virtue approach provides a robust framework for developing such an approach. While public and service users may no longer trust nurses to have all the relevant information, they should be able to trust nurses to act ethically. If this is to be the basis of the trust relationship between nurses and users of their services, then the profession will need to pay close attention to developing ethical practice and decision making not only in the initial stages of professional education but also in life-long learning and practice. The profession itself will have to maintain an overview of ethical standards and be ready to act to support such standards.

As we noted in Chapter 1, the 1990s can be characterised in health services as the risk decade. However, risk was defined in a narrow technical fashion, as threat and danger, and the role of nurses was interpreted as that of a hazard manager. As we move into the new millennium, risk will remain important, but if we are to use it creatively to empower users and nurses, then we must move beyond the technical and incorporate ethics into our understanding of risk. Risk must be defined broadly and nurses must manage risk creatively, balancing threats and opportunities.

REFERENCES

Adams, J. (1995) *Risk.* UCL Press, London.

Alaszewski, A. and Manthorpe, J. (1991) Measuring and managing risk in social welfare. *British Journal of Social Work,* **21,** 277–90.

Alaszewski, A. and Manthorpe, J. (1993) Quality and the welfare services: a literature review. *British Journal of Social Work,* **23,** 653–66.

Alaszewski, A., Alaszewski, H., Manthorpe, J. and Ayer, S. (1998a) *Assessing and managing risk in nursing education and practice: supporting vulnerable people in the community.* Research report Series 10. English National Board for Nursing, Midwifery and Health Visiting, London.

Alaszewski, A., Harrison, L. and Manthorpe, J. (eds) (1998b) *Risk, Health and Welfare: Policies, Strategies and Practices.* Open University Press, Buckingham.

Alberg, C., Hatfield, B. and Huxley, P. (1996) *Learning Materials on Mental Health: Risk Assessment.* The University of Manchester and the Department of Health, Manchester.

Almond, B. (2000) Commodifying animals: ethical issues in genetic engineering of animals. *Health, Risk and Society,* **2**(1), 95–105.

Atkinson, D. and Williams, F. (eds) (1990) *'Know me as I am': An Anthology of Prose, Poetry and Art by People with Learning Difficulties.* Hodder and Stoughton, London.

Ayto, J. (1990) *Dictionary of Word Origins.* Bloomsbury, London.

Barnes, D. (1997) *Older People with Mental Health Problems Living Alone: Anybody's Priority?* Department of Health, London.

Beck, U. (1992) *Risk Society: Towards a New Modernity.* Sage, London.

Benner, P. (1984) *From Novice to Expert: Excellence and Power in Clinical Nursing Practice.* Addison-Wesley, Menlo Park, California.

Bennett, P. and Calman, K. (1999) Pulling the threads together. In: Bennett, P. and Calman, K. (eds) *Risk Communication and Public Health.* Oxford University Press, Oxford.

Bentham, J. (1982) *An Introduction to the Principles of Morals and Legislation.* Methuen, London.

Bernstein, P.L. (1996) *Against the Gods: The Remarkable Story of Risk.* John Wiley and Sons, New York.

Booth, T.A. (1981) Collaboration between health and social services. *Policy and Politics,* **9,** 23–49 and 205–26.

Borrill, J. and Bird, L. (1999) *All about Anxiety.* The Mental Health Foundation, London.

Boseley, S. (1999a) Chaos reigned at baby heart centre. The *Guardian,* Wednesday 17 March 1999, p. 6.

Boseley, S. (1999b) Father 'given false information' over girl's operation. The *Guardian,* Thursday 18 March 1999, p. 6.

Boyd, W. (chair) (1996) *Report of the confidential inquiry into homicides and suicides by mentally ill people.* Royal College of Psychiatrists, London.

Brooker, C., Davies, S., Ellis, L. *et al.* (1997) *Promoting Autonomy and Independence among Older People: An Evaluation of Educational Programmes in Nursing.* English National Board for Nursing, Midwifery and Health Visiting, London.

Bucknall, T. and Thomas, S. (1997) Nurses' reflection on problems associated with decision-making in critical care settings. *Journal of Advanced Nursing,* **25,** 229–37.

Butler-Sloss Inquiry (1988) *Report of the Inquiry into Child Sexual Abuse in Cleveland 1987, Presented to the Secretary of State for Social Services by the Right Honourable Lord Butler-Sloss DBE,* Cm 412. HMSO, London.

Bytheway, B. (1995) *Ageism.* Open University Press, Buckingham.

Calman, K.C., Bennett, P.G. and Coles, D.G. (1999) Risks to health: some issues in management, regulation and communication. *Health, Risk and Society,* **1,** 107–16.

Checkland, P. and Scholes, P. (1990) *Soft Systems Methodology in Action.* John Wiley and Sons, Chichester.

Checkland, S.G. and Checkland, E.O.A. (eds) (1974) *The Poor Law Report of 1834.* Penguin, Harmondsworth.

Cioffi, J. (1997) Heuristics, servants to intuition, in clinical decision-making. *Journal of Advanced Nursing,* **26,** 203–7.

Clarke, C. and Heyman, B. (1998) Risk management for people with dementia. In: Heyman, B. (ed.) *Risk, Health and Health Care: A Qualitative Approach.* Arnold, London.

Cohen, S. (1972) *Folk Devils and Moral Panics: The creation of the Mods and Rockers.* MacGibbon and Kee, London.

Coombes, R. (1999) UKCC and national boards to be axed. *Nursing Times*, **95**(6), 10 February, p. 5.

Cook, C. and Easthope, G. (1996) Symptoms of a crises? Trust, risk and medicine: review essay. *Australian and New Zealand Journal of Sociology*, **32**(3), 85–98.

Coote, A. (1998) Risk and public policy: towards a high-trust democracy. In: Franklin, J. (ed.) *The Politics of Risk Society*. Polity Press, Cambridge.

Corby, B. (1993) *Child Abuse: Towards a Knowledge Base*. Open University Press, Buckingham.

Corby, B. (1996) Risk assessment in child protection work. In: Kemshall, H. and Pritchard, J. (eds) *Good Practice in Risk Assessment and Risk Management*. Jessica Kingsley, London.

Corkish, C. and Heyman, B. (1998) The resettlement of people with severe learning difficulties. In: Heyman, B. (ed.) *Risk, Health and Health Care*. Arnold, London.

Cox, D., Crossland, B., Darby, S.C. *et al.* (1992) Estimations of risk from observations on humans. In: the Royal Society (ed.) *Risk, Analysis, Perception and Management: Report of a Royal Society Study Group*. The Royal Society, London.

Cunningham-Burley, S. and Kerr, A. (1999) Special issue on risk and the new genetics. *Health, Risk and Society*, **1**.

Daily Telegraph (1998) Care before community, Editorial. The *Daily Telegraph*, 17 January 1998, p. 25.

Dawson, S. (1992) *Analysing Organisations*, 2nd edn. Macmillan Press, London.

Department of Health and Social Security (1973) *Collaboration between NHS and Local Government: A Report from the Working Party*. DHSS, London.

Department of Health and Social Security (1982) *Child Abuse: A Study of Inquiry Reports, 1973–1981*, HMSO, London.

Department of Health and Social Security (1986) *Child Abuse – Working Together, A Draft Guide to Arrangements for Interagency Co-operation for the Protection of Children*. DHSS, London.

Department of Health (1995) *The Patient's Charter and You*. Department of Health, London.

Department of Health, the Scottish Office and the Welsh Office (1996) *The Obligations of Care*. HMSO, London.

Department of Health (1997a) *The Health of the Nation: Briefing Pack*. http://www.open.gov.uk/doh/hon97.

Department of Health (1997b) *The New NHS*, Cm 3807. The Stationery Office, London.

Department of Health (1998a) *Our Healthier Nation: A Contract for Health*, Cm 3852. The Stationery Office, London.

Department of Health (1998b) *A First Class Service*. Department of Health, London.

Department of Health (1999) *Saving Lives: Our Healthier Nation*, Cm 4386. The Stationery Office, London.

Department of Trade and Industry (1990) *Home and Leisure Accident Research: 12th Annual Report of the Home Accident Surveillance System*. Department of Trade and Industry, London.

Dobos, C. (1992) Defining risk from the perspective of nurses in clinical roles. *Journal of Advanced Nursing*, **17**, 1303–9.

Doubilet, P. and McNeil, B.J. (1988) Clinical decision making. In: Dowie, J. and Elstein, A. (eds) *Professional Judgment: A Reader in Clinical Decision Making*. Cambridge University Press, Cambridge.

Douglas, M. (1990) Risk as a forensic resource risk. *Dædalus, Journal of the American Academy of Arts and Sciences*, **119**, 1–16.

Dowie, J. (1999) Communication for better decisions: not about risk. *Health, Risk and Society*, **1**, 41–53.

Dowie, J. and Elstein, A. (1988a) Introduction. In: Dowie, J. and Elstein, A. (eds) *Professional Judgment: A Reader in Clinical Decision Making*. Cambridge University Press, Cambridge.

Dowie, J. and Elstein, A. (eds) (1988b) *Professional Judgment: A Reader in Clinical Decision Making*. Cambridge University Press, Cambridge.

Downie, R. (1989) What should be the limits of paternalism? What rights do society's professionals have to interfere?, In: *Rights, Risks and Responsibilities, The Proceedings of the Conference held at St. Andrew's College of Education Bearsdon*. Age Concern Scotland, Edinburgh.

Duffield, C. (1991) Maintaining competence for the first-line nurse managers; an evaluation of the use of the literature. *Journal of Advanced Nursing*, **16**, 55–62.

Durkheim, E. (1952) In: Simpson, G. (ed.) *Suicide: A Study in Sociology*. Routledge and Kegan Paul, London.

Eddy, D.M. (1988) Variations in physician practice: the role of uncertainty. In: Dowie, J. and Elstein, A. (eds) *Professional Judgment: A Reader in Clinical Decision Making*. Cambridge University Press, Cambridge.

Elstein, A.S., Holzman, G.B., Ravitch, M.M. *et al.* (1988) Comparison of physicians' decisions regarding estrogen replacement women therapy for menopausal women and decisions derived from a decision analytic model. In: Dowie, J. and Elstein, A. (eds) *Professional Judgment: A Reader in Clinical Decision Making.* Cambridge University Press, Cambridge.

ENB (1997) Promoting autonomy and independence among older people: an evaluation of educational programmes in nursing. *Research Highlights, 27.* English National Board for Nursing, Midwifery and Health Visiting, London.

Erlen, J.A. and Sereika, S.M. (1997) Critical care nurses, ethical decision-making. *Journal of Advanced Nursing,* **26**, 953–61.

Evans-Pritchard, E.E. (1937) *Witchcraft, Oracles and Magic among the Azande.* Clarendon Press, Oxford.

Faludi, A. (1973) *Planning Theory.* Pergamon Press, Oxford.

Fletcher, S. (1991) *NVQs: Standards and Competence: A Practical Guide for Employers, Managers and Trainers.* Kogan Page, London.

Franklin, B. (1999) *Hard Pressed: National Newspapaer Reporting of Social Work and Social Services.* Reed Business Press, Sutton, Surrey.

Freeman, M.D.A. (1994) Legislating for child abuse. In: Levy, A. (ed.) *Refocus on Child Abuse: Medical, Legal and Social Perspectives.* Hawksmere, London.

Friend, J.K., Power, J.M. and Yewlett, C.S.L. (1974) *Public Planning: The Intercorporate Dimension.* Tavistock, London.

Fruin, D. (1998) *Moving into Mainstream: The Report of a National Inspection of Services for Adults with Learning Disabilities.* Department of Health, Social Care Group, SSI.

Gherardi, S. (1999) Man-made disasters 20 years on: critical commentary. *Health, Risk and Society,* **1**, 233–9.

Gibson, M.J. (1990) Falls in later life. In: Kane, R.L., Grimley Evans, J. and MacFayden, D. (eds), *Improving the Health of Older People: A World View.* Oxford University Press, Oxford.

Giddens, A. (1990) *The Consequences of Modernity.* Polity Press, Cambridge.

Giddens, A. (1991) *Modernity and Self-Identity: Self and Society in the Late Modern Society.* Polity Press, Cambridge.

Gilbert, T. (1998) Towards a politics of trust. *Journal of Advanced Nursing,* **27**, 1010–16.

Glennerster, H., Korman, N. and Marslen-Wilson, F. (1983a) *Planning for Priority Groups.* Martin Richardson, Oxford.

Glennerster, H., Korman, N. and Marslen-Wilson, F. (1983b) Plans and practice: the participants' views. *Public Administration,* **61**, 265–81.

Goffman, E. (1968) *Stigma: Notes on the Management of Spoiled Identity.* Penguin, Harmondsworth.

Green, J. (1999) From accidents to risk: public health and preventable injury. *Health, Risk and Society,* **1**, 25–39.

The *Guardian* (1998a) Handicapped man lost in Majorca. The *Guardian,* 29 September 1998, p. 5.

The *Guardian* (1998b) Four die as canal boat sinks – disabled trippers trapped after narrow boat is snagged in lock. The *Guardian,* 20 August 1998, p. 5.

The *Guardian* (1998c) Care centre grieves as victims of narrow boat accident named. The *Guardian,* 21 August 1998, p. 10.

Hallett, C. (1995) *Interagency Coordination in Child Protection, Studies in Child Protection.* HMSO, London.

Hallowell, N. (1999) Advising on the management of genetic risk: offering choice or prescribing action? *Health, Risk and Society,* **1**, 267–80.

Hamm, R.M. (1988) Clinical expertise and the cognitive continuum. In: Dowie, J. and Elstein, A. (eds) *Professional Judgment: A Reader in Clinical Decision Making.* Cambridge University Press, Cambridge.

Hanlon, G. (1998) Professionalism as enterprise: service class politics and the redefinition of professionalism. *Sociology,* **32**, 43–63.

Harrison, L. and Tether, P. (1987) The co-ordination of UK policy on alcohol and tobacco. *Policy and Politics,* **15**, 77–90.

Hayward, J. (1975) *Information: a Prescription against Pain.* Study of Nursing Care Project. Reports: series 2; No. 5, Royal College of Nursing, London.

Healt Act (1999). The Stationery Office, London.

Helman, C.G. (1994) *Culture, Health and Illness: An Introduction for Health Professionals,* 3rd edn. Butterworth-Heinemann, Oxford.

Heyman, B. and Henricksen, M. (1998) Probability and health risks. In: Heyman, B. (ed.) *Risk, Health and Health Care: A Qualitative Approach.* Arnold, London.

Heyman, B. and Huckle, S. (1993) Not worth the risk? Attitudes of adults with learning difficulties, and their informal carers to the hazards of everyday life. *Social Science and Medicine*, **37**, 1557–64.

Heyman, B., Huckle, S. and Handyside E.C. (1998) Freedom of the locality for people with learning difficulties. In: Heyman, B. (ed.) *Risk, Health and Health Care: A qualitative approach*. Arnold, London.

Holm, D. and Stephenson, S. (1994) Reflection: a student's perspective. In: Palmer, A.M., Burnes, S. and Bulman, C. (eds) *Reflective Practice in Nursing: The Growth of the Professional Practitioner*. Blackwell, London.

Hood, C.C., Jones, D.K.C., Pidgeon, N.F., Turner, B.A. and Gibson, R. (1992) Risk Management. In: the Royal Society (ed.) *Risk, Analysis, Perception and Management: Report of a Royal Society Study Group*. The Royal Society, London.

Hudson, B. (1999a) Primary health care and social care: working across professional boundaries, part one: the changing context of inter-professional relationships. *Managing Community Care*, **7**, 15–22.

Hudson, B. (1999b) Primary health care and social care: working across professional boundaries, part two: models of inter-professional collaboration. *Managing Community Care*, **7**(2), 15–20.

Husted, G.L. and Husted, J.M. (1995) *Ethical Decision Making in Nursing*, 2nd edn. Mosby, St. Louis.

Jay Committee (1979) *Report of the Committee of Enquiry into Mental Handicap Nursing and Care*, Chairman Peggy Jay, Vol 1, Cmnd 7468–1. HMSO, London.

Jeffrey, C. (1998) Speaking out. *Nursing Times*, **94**(50), 21; 16 December.

Johns, C. (1994) Guided reflection. In: Palmer, A.M., Burnes, S. and Bulman, C. (eds) *Reflective Practice in Nursing: The Growth of the Professional Practitioner*. Blackwell, London.

Kitzinger, J. (1999) Researching risk and the media. *Health, Risk and Society*, **1**, 55–69.

Klein, K. and Pauker, S.G. (1988) Recurrent deep venous thrombosis in pregnancy: analysis of the risks and benefits of anticoagulation. In: Dowie, J. and Elstein, A. (eds) *Professional Judgment: A Reader in Clinical Decision Making*. Cambridge University Press, Cambridge.

Lankshear, A., Brown, J. and Thompson, C. (1996) *Mapping the Nursing Competencies Required in Institutional and Community Settings in the Context of Multidisciplinary Care Provision: An Exploratory Study*. English National Board, London.

Leach, E.R. (1957) The epistemological background to Malinowski's empiricism. In: Firth, R. (ed.) *Man & Culture: An Evaluation of the Work of Bronislaw Malinowski*. Routledge and Kegan Paul, London.

Lindblom, C.E. (1965) *The Intelligence of Democracy*. Free Press, New York.

Lindblom, C.E. (1979) Still muddling, not yet through. *Public Administration Review*, **39**, 517–25.

Lippman, A. (1999) Choice as a risk to women's health. *Health, Risk and Society*, **1**, 281–91.

Luker, K.A. and Kenrick, M. (1992) An exploratory study of the sources of influence on the clinical decisions of community nurses. *Journal of Advanced Nursing*, **17**, 457–66.

Lupton, D. (1999) *Risk*. Routledge, London.

Lyon, C.M. and de Cruz, P. (1993) *Child Abuse*, 2nd edn. Family Law, Bristol.

MacDonald, M. (1984) Natural Rights. In: Waldron, J. (ed.) *Theories of Rights*. Oxford University Press, Oxford.

McInnes, M. (1989) Chairman's introduction. In: *Rights, Risks and Responsibilities, The Proceedings of the Conference held at St. Andrew's College of Education Bearsdon*. Age Concern Scotland, Edinburgh.

MacIntyre, A. (1967) *A Short History of Ethics*. Routledge and Kegan Paul, London.

McKeganey, N. and Hunter, D. (1986) Only connect … tightrope walking and joint working in the care of the elderly. *Policy and Politics*, **14**, 335–60.

Means, R. and Smith, R. (1994) *Community Care: Policy and Practice*. Macmillan, London.

Menzies, I.E.P. (1970) *The functioning of social systems as a defence against anxiety: a report on a study of the nursing service of a general hospital*. Tavistock Institute of Human Relations, London.

Millar, B. (1999) Clinical governance: Carry that weight. *Health Service Journal*, 18 February 1999, pp. 22–27.

Munro, E.M. (1999) Protecting children in an anxious society. *Health, Risk and Society*, **1**, 117–27.

Myers, F. and MacDonald, C. (1996) 'I was given options not choices': involving older users and carers in assessment and care planning. In: Bland, R. (ed.) *Developing Services for Older People and Their Families*. Jessica Kingsley, London.

Narayan, S.M. and Corcoran-Perry, S. (1997) Lines of reasoning as a representation of nurses' clinical decision making. *Research in Nursing and Health*, **20**, 353–64.

National Confidential Inquiry (1999) *Safer Services*. National Confidential Inquiry into Suicide and Homicide by People with Mental Illness, London.

NHS Executive (1999) *Clinical governance: in the new NHS*. Health Service Circular, HSC 1999/065, Department of Health, Leeds.

Nirje, B. (1972) The right to self-determination. In: Wolfensberger, W. with Nirje, B., Olansky, S., Perske, R. and Roos, P. *The Principles of Normalization in Human Services*. National Institute on Mental Retardation through Leonard Crainford, Toronto.

The Nurses, Midwives and Health Visitors (Registered Fever Nurses Amendment Rules and Training Amendment Rules) Approval Order (1989) No. 1456.

Offerdy, M. (1998) The application of decision making concepts by nurse practitioners in general practice. *Journal of Advanced Nursing*, **28**, 988–1000.

Paine, T. (1921) *Rights of Man*. Dent, London.

Palmer, A.M. Burnes, S. and Bulman, C. (eds) (1994) *Reflective Practice in Nursing*. Blackwell, London.

Parsons, T. (1951) *The Social System*. Routledge and Kegan Paul, London.

Parsons, T. (1966) Professions. In: Sills, D.L. (ed.) *International Encyclopedia of the Social Sciences*, Volume 12. Macmillan and the Free Pres, New York.

Parton, N. (1999) Ideology, Politics and Policy. In: Stevenson, O. (ed.) *Child Welfare in the UK*. Blackwell, Oxford.

Pearsall, J. (ed.) (1998) *The New Oxford Dictionary of English*. Clarendon Press, Oxford.

Perske, R. (1972) The dignity of risk. In: Wolfensberger, W. with Nirje, B., Olansky, S., Perske, R. and Roos, P. *The Principles of Normalization in Human Services*. National Institute on Mental Retardation through Leonard Crainford, Toronto.

Peterborough CVS (1997) *Peterborough Voices: Extraordinary People, Extraordinary Lives*. Peterborough Council for Voluntary Services, Peterborough.

Petersen, A. (1999) Counselling the genetically 'at risk': a critique of 'non-directiveness. *Health, Risk and Society*, **1**, 253–65.

Pietzner, C. (1990) *A Candle on the Hill: Images of Camphill Life*. Floris Books, Edinburgh.

Plant, R. (1991) *Modern Political Thought*. Basil Blackwell, Oxford.

Pritchard, J. (1997) Vulnerable people taking risks: older people and residential care. In: Kemshall, H. and Pritchard, J. (eds) *Good Practice in Risk and Risk Management 2, Protection, Rights and Responsibilities*. Jessica Kingsley, London.

Rawls, J. (1972) *A Theory of Justice*. Oxford University Press, Oxford.

Reder, P., Duncan, S. and Gray, M. (1993) *Beyond Blame: Child Abuse Tragedies Revisited*. Routledge, London.

Reed, J. (1998) Care and protection for older people. In: Heyman, B. (ed.) *Risk, Health and Health Care: A Qualitative Approach*. Arnold, London.

Reith, M. (1998) *Community Care Tragedies*. Venture Press, Birmingham.

Rhodes, R.A.W. (1987) Mrs Thatcher and local government: intentions and achievements. In: Robins, L. (ed.) *Political Institutions in Britain: Development and Change*. Longman, London.

Ritchie Report (1994) *The Report of the Inquiry into the Care and Treatment of Christopher Clunis* (Chairman, J.H. Ritchie). HMSO, London.

Ryan, T. (ed.) (1999) *Managing Crisis and Risk in Mental Health Nursing*. Stanley Thornes, Cheltenham.

Saunders, M. (1999) *Managing Risk in Services for People with a Learning Disability*. APLD Publications, Nottingham.

Scally, G. and Donaldson, L.J. (1998) Clinical governance and the drive for quality improvement in the new NHS in England. *British Medical Journal*, **317**, 61–5.

Schön, D.A. (1988) From technical rationality to reflection-in-action. In: Dowie, J. and Elstein, A. (eds) *Professional Judgment, a Reader in Clinical Decision Making*. Cambridge University Press, Cambridge.

Schön, D.A. (1991) *The Reflective Practitioner*, 2nd edn. Temple Smith, London.

Schutz, A. (1971) *Collected Papers, Volume 1, The Problem of Social Reality*. Nijhoff, the Hague.

Scott, H. (1998) Risk and community care for people with mental illness. In: Heyman, B. (ed.) *Risk, Health and Health Care*. Arnold, London.

Secretary of State for Social Services (1974) *Report of the Committee of Inquiry into the Care and Supervision Provided in Relation to Maria Colwell*. HMSO, London.

Semple, J. (1993) *Bentham's Prison: A Study of the Panopticon Penitentiary*. Clarendon Press, Oxford.

Shearer, A. (1980) *Handicapped Children in Residential Care: A Study of Policy Failure.* Bedford Square Press, London.

Simpson, J.A. and Weiner, E.S.C. (eds) (1989) *The Oxford English Dictionary*, 2nd edn. Clarendon Press, Oxford.

Skeet, M.H. (1970) *Home from Hospital: A Study of the Home Care Needs of Recently Discharged Patients.* Dan Mason Nursing Research Committee, London.

Sletteboe A. (1997) Dilemma: a conceptual analysis. *Journal of Advanced Nursing*, **26**, 449–54.

Smith, G. and Cantley, C. (1985) *Assessing Health Care: A Study in Organisational Evaluation.* Open University Press, Milton Keynes.

Smith, G. and May, D. (1993) The artificial debate between rationalist and incrementalist models of decision making. In: Hill, M. (ed.) *The Policy Process: A Reader.* Harvester Wheatsheaf, London.

Spencer, K. (1997) If you go down in the woods today ... you certainly don't want to catch Lyme disease. *The Guardian*, Tuesday 11 November 1997, p. 16.

Stanley, N. and Manthorpe, J. (1997) Risk assessment: developing training in mental health work. *Social Work and Social Sciences Review*, **7**, 26–38.

Strang, J. and Farrell, M. (1992) Harm minimisation for drug misusers: when second best may be best first. *British Medical Journal*, **304**, 1127–8.

Sykes, J.B. (ed.) (1982) *The Concise Oxford Dictionary of Current English.* Clarendon Press, Oxford.

Thomson, A. and Sylvester, R. (1998) Care in the Community is scrapped: Dobson pledges more secure units for mentally-ill patients who pose danger. *Daily Telegraph*, 17 January 1998.

Tizard, J. (1964) *Community Services for the Mentally Handicapped.* Oxford University Press, Oxford.

Turner, B.A. and Pidgeon, N.E. (1997) *Man-Made Disasters.* Butterworth-Heinemann, Oxford.

UKCC (1992) *Code of Professional Conduct*, 3rd edn. United Kingdom Central Council for Nursing, Midwifery and Health Visiting, London.

UKCC (1996) *Guidelines for Professional Practice.* United Kingdom Central Council for Nursing, Midwifery and Health Visiting, London.

UKCC (1998) *Guidelines for Mental Health and Learning Disabilities Nursing.* United Kingdom Central Council for Nursing, Midwifery and Health Visiting, London.

UKCC (1999) *How the UKCC Works for You: Protecting the Public through Professional Standards.* United Kingdom Central Council for Nursing, Midwifery and Health Visiting, London.

Vincent, C. (1997) Risk, safety and the dark side of quality: improving quality in health care should include removing the causes of harm. *British Medical Journal*, **314**, 1775–6.

Waldron, J. (1984) Introduction. In: Waldron, J. (ed.) *Theories of Rights.* Oxford University Press, Oxford.

Warner, Sir Fredrick (1992) Introduction. In: *Risk: analysis, perception and management.* Report of a Royal Society Study Group, The Royal Society, London.

Warnock, M. (1998) *An Intelligent Person's Guide to Ethics.* Duckworth, London.

Wharton, F. (1992) Risk management: basic concepts and general principles. In: Ansell, J. and Wharton, F. (eds) *Risk: Analysis, Assessment and Management.* John Wiley and Sons, Chichester.

Wildavsky, A. (1979) *The Art and Craft of Policy Analysis.* Macmillan, Basingstoke.

Williamson, J. (1989) Falls in old age. In: *Rights, Risks and Responsibilities, The Proceedings of the Conference held at St. Andrew's College of Education Bearsdon.* Age Concern Scotland, Edinburgh.

Wistow, G. and Fuller, S. (1983) *Joint Planning in Perspective, the National Association of Health Authorities, the NAHA Survey of Collaboration, 1976–1982.* Loughbourough University, Centre for Research in Social Policy, Loughborough.

Wolfensberger, W. (1972) Dignity and risk: a further reflection. In: Wolfensberger, W. with Nirje, B., Olansky, S., Perske, R. and Roos, P. *The Principles of Normalization in Human Services.* National Institute on Mental Retardation through Leonard Crainford, Toronto.

Wright, F. with Whyley, C. (1994) *Accident Prevention and Risk-Taking by Elderly People: The Need for Advice.* Age Concern Institute of Gerontology, King's College, London.

Wyatt, J. (1998) Four barriers to realising the information revolution in health care. In: Lenaghan, J. (ed.) *Rethinking IT and Health.* Institute for Public Policy Research, London.

Young, K. (1977) Values in the policy processes. *Policy and Politics*, **5**, 3.

Zimmerman, D.H. and Wieder, D.L. (1977) The diary-interview method. *Urban Life*, **5**(4), 479–89.

Index